How Iran's Duplicitous Diplomacy, Callous Policies Cost Lives

A Report on the COVID-19 Crisis

Published by

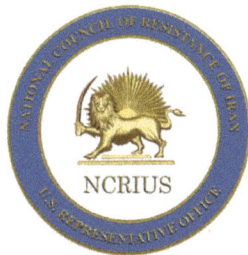

NCRIUS

NATIONAL COUNCIL OF RESISTANCE OF IRAN
U.S. REPRESENTATIVE OFFICE (NCRI-US)

How Iran's Duplicitous Diplomacy, Callous Policies Cost Lives
A Report on the COVID-19 Crisis

First published in 2020 by
National Council of Resistance of Iran — U.S. Representative Office (NCRI-US),
1747 Pennsylvania Ave., NW, Suite 1125, Washington, DC 20006

ISBN-10 (paperback): 1-944942-38-6
ISBN-13 (paperback): 978-1-944942-38-0
ISBN-10 (e-book): 1-944942-39-4
ISBN-13 (e-book): 978-1-944942-39-7

Library of Congress Control Number: 2020936619

Library of Congress Cataloging-in-Publication Data

National Council of Resistance of Iran — U.S. Representative Office.

How Iran's Duplicitous Diplomacy, Callous Policies Cost Lives

1. Iran. 2. Coronavirus. 3. Corruption. 4. Human Rights. 5. COVID-19

First Edition: April 2020
Second Edition: May 2020
Printed in the United States of America

Table of Contents

Executive Summary 5

The Regime's Offensive Against Sanctions 9

Facts Speak Louder Than Words .13

Official U.S. Position 17

Terrorism Overrides Healthcare 23

Theft and Hoarding of Medical Resources 25

The Iranian People's Wealth in the Hands of Khamenei
and the IRGC 31

Khamenei and Rouhani Sending People Back to Work
at the Height of the Pandemic 41

Attacking Americans in Iraq to Divert Attention Away
from the Coronavirus Crisis 43

Conclusion 47

Appendix I 53

Appendix II 63

Appendix III 73

List of publications 77

About the NCRI-US 83

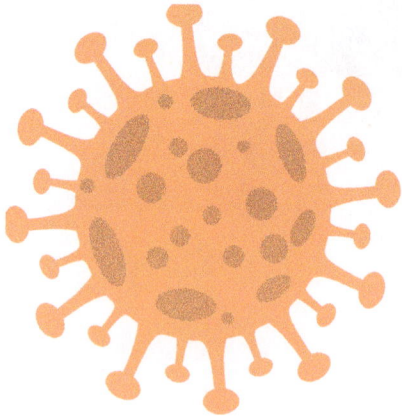

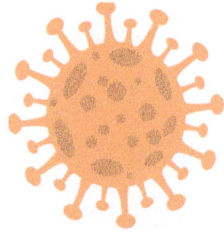

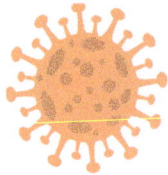

Executive Summary

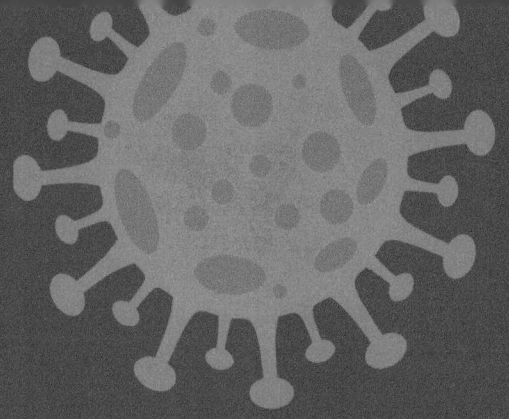

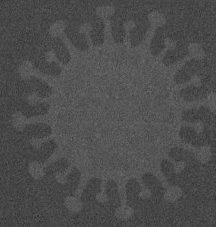

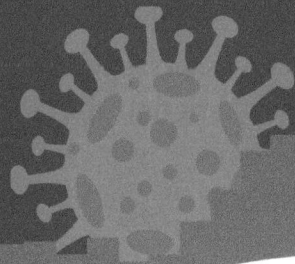

The coronavirus pandemic has morphed into a global crisis, with virtually the entire international community resisting its onslaught. Governments around the world have leveraged all resources at their disposal to protect their citizens from a virus that threatens everyone.

But the situation is different with regard to the regime ruling Iran, whose conduct confirms it has no regard for the pain, suffering and deaths of the Iranian people. Instead, the theocracy views this catastrophe as a political opportunity that it can exploit in its domestic and foreign policies. Which explains why, despite knowing about the outbreak and spread of the virus in Iran, it ignored warnings and deliberately misled the public to prevent the virus from impacting its orchestrated February 11 anniversary festivities and the February 21st sham parliamentary elections.

As the coronavirus began to wreak havoc in many countries, and the number of fatalities and infections spiked in Iran, the regime launched a massive international campaign advocating the lifting of the sanctions imposed due to its terrorism, human rights violations and nuclear weapons program. While this orchestrated campaign is playing out on the world stage, inside Iran the regime tries to downplay the number of fatalities.

To advance its objective, the regime claims that international sanctions are the root cause of Iran's lack of medical resources and equipment, as well as treatment options and pharmaceuticals. These claims, intended to create cracks in the wall of sanctions, are demonstrably false.

First, the problem is not a lack of money or resources. Hundreds of billions of dollars of the Iranian people's national wealth are under the control of Supreme Leader Ali Khamenei and the Islamic Revolutionary Guard Corps (IRGC). Even a small percentage of this wealth, if spent on fighting the coronavirus pandemic, could address all of the logistical, resourcing, and healthcare requirements.

Second, the necessary medical equipment and supplies have been hoarded and stored in warehouses by regime-related entities, in order to sell them at radically inflated costs to desperate consumers.

Third, no individual, official or government in the world has imposed sanctions on medical treatment, medical equipment or any related product. On the contrary, the World Health Organization has officially announced that it is prepared to help Iran with any such requirements. U.S. officials have also repeatedly declared that not only are there no sanctions in these areas, but that they also stand ready to provide support.

And finally, Iranian regime officials, including its president, Hassan Rouhani, have stated on the record that the regime has no deficiencies when it comes to healthcare. Officials even boast about exporting or donating medical products to other countries.

This report seeks to show that the Iranian Foreign Ministry's campaign to lift sanctions is replete with lies and misleading claims, with the goal of cynically exploiting the coronavirus pandemic to the regime's benefit. In effect, the mullahs are causing the death of thousands of Iranians to preserve their own rule. The correct policy is not to give in to this campaign, but rather to pressure the regime to unleash the available resources that belong to the Iranian people and that are urgently needed to combat the human tragedy unfolding in Iran—a tragedy aggravated by regime corruption and mismanagement. If other countries and international organizations want to assist the Iranian people, they should not provide resources to the regime; rather, they should dedicate their assistance to the World Health Organization, which can then release it directly to the oppressed people of Iran.

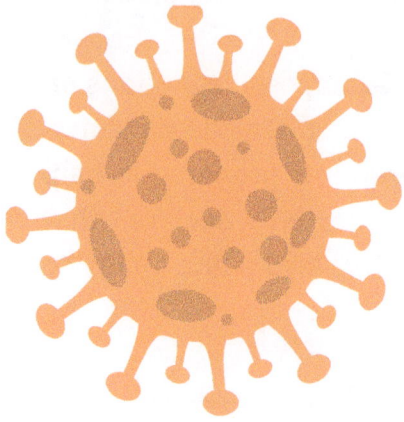

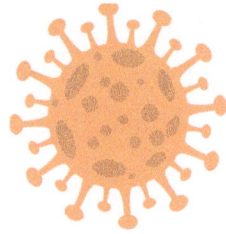

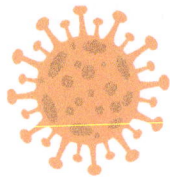

The Regime's Offensive Against Sanctions

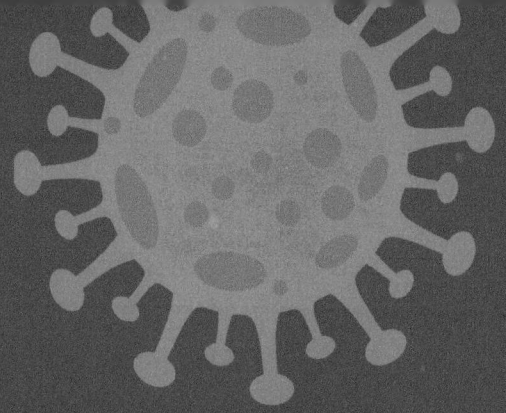

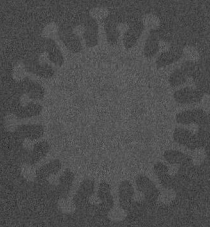

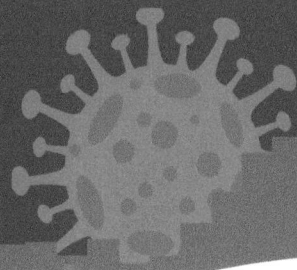

Foreign Minister Mohammad-Javad Zarif wrote a letter on March 12 to the UN Secretary General, containing a number of lies about the lack of resources to prevent and confront the coronavirus in Iran and adding that it is "imperative that the government of the United States immediately ... lift all sanctions it has illegally imposed on my country."[1]

According to the regime's state media, in addition to contacting the UN Secretary General, Zarif has also spoken on the phone with over 25 foreign ministers in the context of "coronavirus diplomacy." He urged all of them to leverage their political and diplomatic resources to lift sanctions against the regime.[2]

Zarif's subordinates have also been active in using the pandemic as a cover to lift sanctions. The Iranian regime's envoy to the United Nations, Majid Takht Ravanchi, has called on other countries to "defy sanctions" if the U.S. ignores the requests of governments and UN officials to lift sanctions against the clerical regime. Why? He explains: "So we can more effectively fight against COVID-19."[3]

Ten days prior to that, Ravanchi had tweeted: "People and government of Iran working hard to defeat #Covid_19, but US sanctions impeding their efforts".[4]

His colleague, Hamid Baeidinejad, the regime's ambassador to the United Kingdom, is also active in this campaign, using methods typically reserved for opposition activists, including petitions signed by British citizens asking for the lifting of sanctions. The state-run website Tabnak wrote on March 26, 2020: "Baeidinejad, Iran's ambassador in London, has announced that as of today, 12,824 people in Britain have signed a petition calling on the U.S. government to lift sanctions against Iran during the period it confronts the coronavirus."

The speaker of the regime's parliament (*Majlis*), Ali Larijani, has also sent multiple letters to the President of the Inter-Parliamentary Union, the Secretary General of the Union of Parliaments of member states of the Organization of Islamic

---

1   Iranian Students' News Agency (ISNA News Agency, March 12, 2020), https://bit.ly/39MN7RI

2   Tabnak, March 26, 2020, https://bit.ly/2yFXHxc

3   Iran Students' News Agency (ISNA News Agency, March 25, 2020), https://bit.ly/2UHWsWI

4   Takht Ravanchi, Majid. Twitter Post. March 13, 2020, 1:34 P.M. https://twitter.com/TakhtRavanchi/status/1238518840679686145

Cooperation, the Secretary General of the Asian Parliamentary Assembly, and speakers of parliaments of Islamic and Asian countries. The letters reiterate the regime's demand to lift sanctions.[5]

Tehran also submitted a request to Azerbaijan, the rotating head of the Non-Aligned Movement (NAM), to issue a statement on behalf of the 120 countries it represents, asking for the lifting of US sanctions against the Iranian regime. The regime's Foreign Ministry spokesman said that the measure failed after "some Arab and Islamic governments, most of whom are our neighbors," intervened against it.[6]

---

5   Islamic Consultative Assembly News Agency, March 10, 2020, https://www.icana.ir/Fa/News/444197

6   Iran Students' News Agency (IRNA News Agency, March 18, 2020), https://bit.ly/39Hl0na

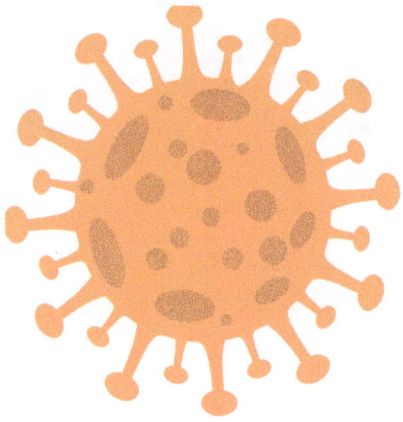

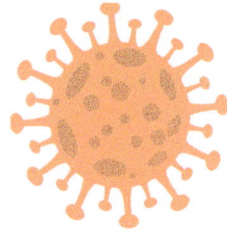

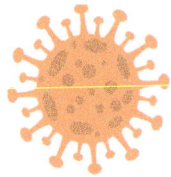

Facts Speak Louder Than Words

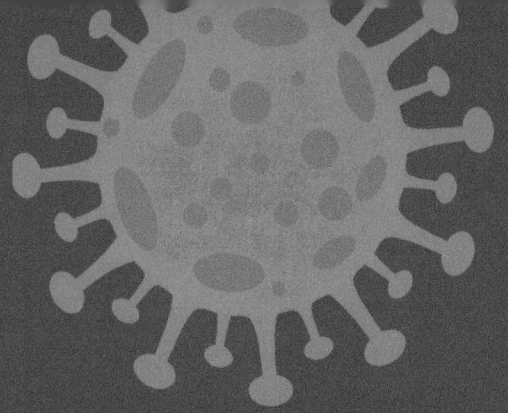

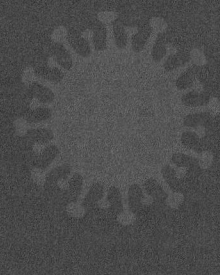

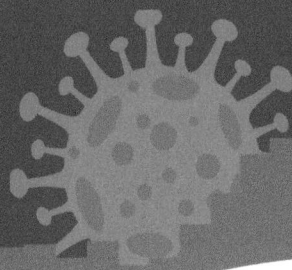

People are dying of the coronavirus in Iran every day, but instead of acting to help them, the clerical regime is inhumanely holding them hostage to advance its policies, particularly the lifting of sanctions. Tehran's lobby in the West and other supporters of the appeasement policy, as well as those who have set their sights on the Iranian market, are coordinating their pro-regime talking points as they shed crocodile tears. They claim that "if we don't help Iran, the country will become the epicenter for the spread of coronavirus, which would be catastrophic for the rest of the world."

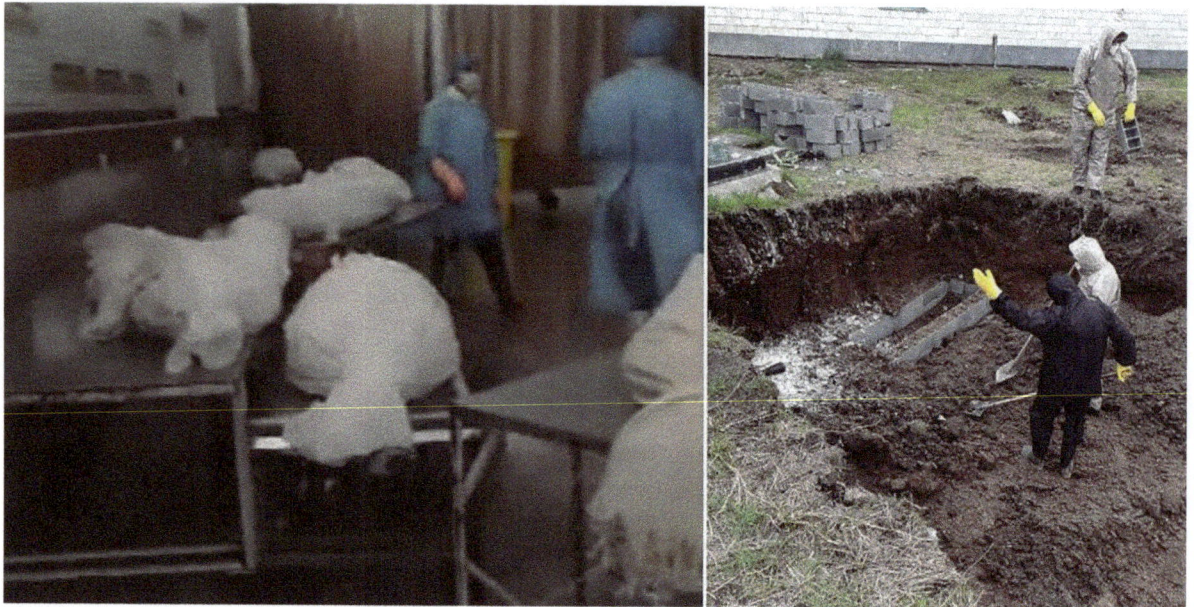

The Observers, France24: The image on the left shows at least 56 body bags awaiting burial at a facility at the main cemetery in Qom. Right: a grave dug for coronavirus victims in Langeroud county in Gilan province, with concrete blocks to separate the bodies.

In fact, the primary murderer of the Iranian people today and the chief reason for the spread of coronavirus resulting in the deaths of over 40,000 Iranians to date, is the regime. A cursory review of the facts reveals the following:

✳ The clerical regime deliberately covered up the coronavirus for three weeks in order to carry out its anniversary celebration and sham elections. The spokesman of Rouhani's cabinet, Ali Rabii, acknowledged that on January 24, when he delivered a letter about coronavirus from the Secretariat of the Public Relations Council to Rouhani, and, in response, Rouhani sounded the alarm on January 26. However, from January 26 to February 19, Rouhani's Health Minister consistently denied any reports about the outbreak of coronavirus in Iran.

* The regime refused to quarantine the city of Qom, one of the epicenters of the spread of the virus in Iran, due to political considerations and its reactionary ideology.

* The IRGC's airliner Mahan Air continued its flights to China even a month after the official declaration of the outbreak in Iran.

* Coronavirus entered Iran directly from China to three cities in Iran. In addition to Qom, where hundreds of Chinese clergies are trained, some of whom were infected, the virus directly went from China to Gilan Province where tourists had gone from China to the Republic of Azerbaijan and from there thru Astara border to Bandar Anzali in Gilan in January 2020. The first cases of corona patients were observed in Gilan in late January. Direct flights of Mahan Air from four Chinese cities to Tehran were the route for the virus to infect the residents in the Capital.

* According to the Health Minister, tens of millions of masks produced were hoarded (by the IRGC and others) and later sold at inflated prices.

* At the height of the spread of the virus, the Secretary General of the Supreme National Security Council provided Iraqi militias (Hashad al-Shaabi) with 50,000 masks as gifts.

* In January, while the regime claimed that it faced financial restrictions as a result of sanctions, it allocated 200 million dollars to the IRGC Qods Force to carry out foreign activities.

* According to a Reuters investigative report, the Setad Foundation, affiliated with Khamenei, has assets valued at roughly 95 billion dollars. According to the US State Department, the office of Supreme Leader Ali Khamenei has assets worth about 200 million dollars. But the regime

refuses to spend any of these assets on the people, although it could without any restrictions work with the WHO and the International Red Cross to allocate some of this wealth to fight coronavirus by procuring medical equipment and drugs for hospitals and average citizens.[7]

* There are more than 10 other organs in Iran controlled by Khamenei, with a total net worth in the hundreds of billions of dollars.

* The regime has refused international assistance, including a US proposal worth a hundred million dollars, but takes Hezbollah terrorists to Iran to fight coronavirus. Many countries, including Kuwait, Azerbaijan, Qatar, Japan, and the European Union, have provided financial aid to the regime without any restrictions.

* A well-equipped medical team from Doctors Without Borders that travelled to the city of Isfahan from France to set up a field hospital were expelled. According to the state-run ISNA news agency on March 25, their program "was completely cancelled." At the same time, an Iranian Health Ministry source said, "If European countries and international organizations want to help the Iranian nation, they must attempt to lift the unjust American sanctions against Iran."[8]

* As Mrs. Maryam Rajavi, the President-elect of the National Council of Resistance of Iran (NCRI) has said, the expulsion of Doctors Without Borders by the regime "is yet another indication that the main problem in Iran is the existence of a corrupt dictatorship that only thinks of preserving its own rule. For them, human lives are worthless. The regime seeks only the assistance that could be put at the disposal of the IRGC and the regime's leaders without any supervision."[9]

---

7   Steve Stecklow, Babak Dehghanpisheh, and Yeganeh Torbati, "Reuters Investigates — Assets of the Ayatollah," Reuters (Thomson Reuters, November 11, 2013), https://www.reuters.com/investigates/iran/#article/part1

8   Iran Students' News Agency, March 25, 2020

9   Rajavi, Maryam. Twitter Post. March 24, 2020, 12:31 P.M. https://twitter.com/Maryam_Rajavi/status/1242489308134567947

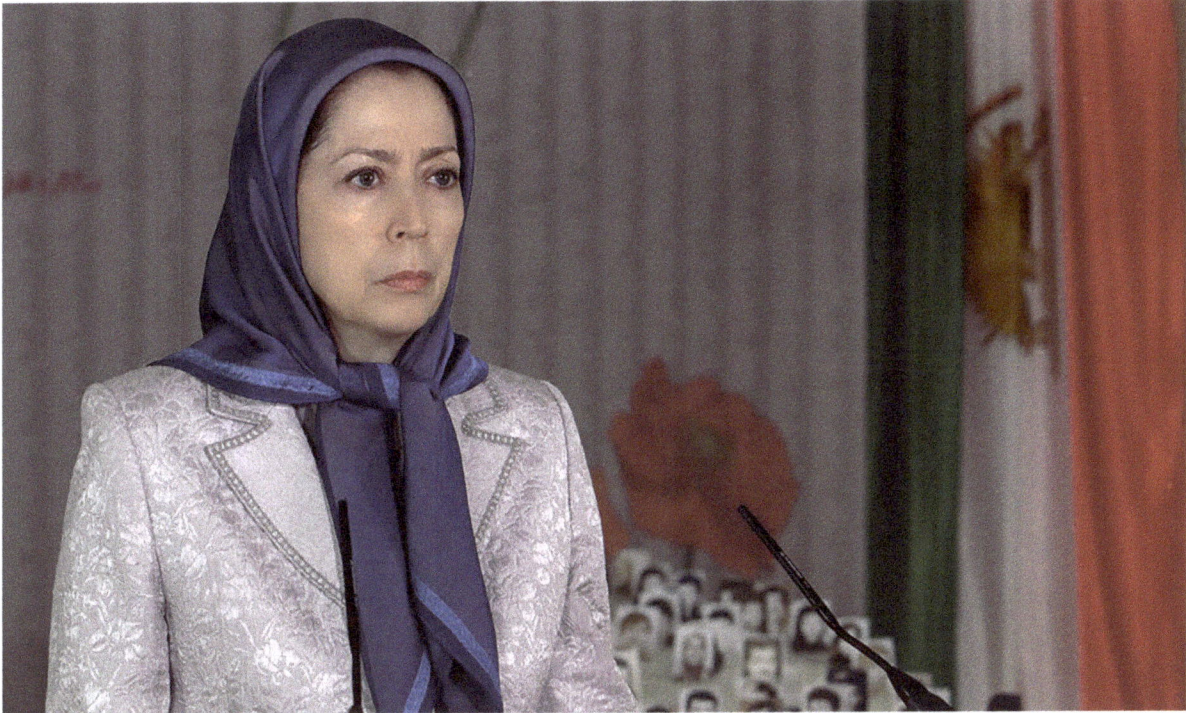

Mrs. Maryam Rajavi, the president-elect of the National Council of Resistance of Iran

✳ On March 27, the French daily *Le Monde* wrote: "A cargo plane containing drugs, medical supplies and sufficient equipment to set up a field hospital with 50 beds for COVID-19 patients at a time when this country suffers from the impacts of the virus is still being held at a hangar at Tehran international airport. ... The equipment was supposed to be used to set up a treatment unit for coronavirus patients in the city of Isfahan, the capital city of one of the worst hit provinces in the country.»[10]

✳ Rouhani has repeatedly claimed that the regime does not have any medical supply shortages and hospital beds remain empty.

✳ The US has officially declared that shipments of medical equipment and drugs to Iran are not sanctioned whatsoever.

An unhinged Khamenei, however, rejected the aid by resorting to conspiracy theories. Alleging that the virus "is specifically built for Iran using the genetic data of Iranians which they have obtained through different means," he said "who in their right mind would trust you to bring them medication? Possibly your medicine is a way to spread the virus more… You might send people as doctors and therapists, maybe they would want to come here and see the effect of the poison they have produced in person."[11]

---

11   John Gambrell, "Iran leader refuses US help, citing virus conspiracy theory," Associated Press, March 22, 2020, https://bit.ly/3aWXnIN

Official U.S. Position

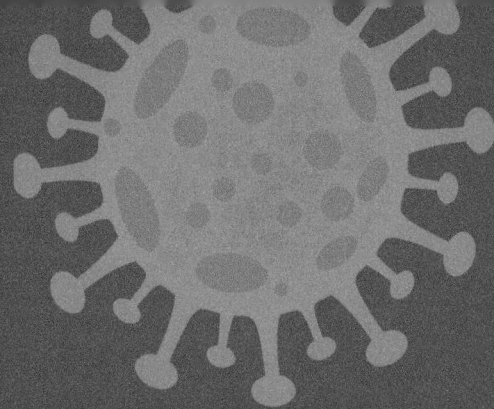

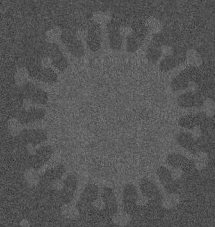

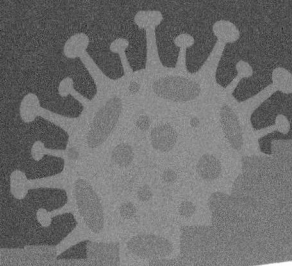

As U.S. authorities have repeatedly made clear, medicine has never been under sanction. The Swiss Ambassador in Tehran announced on January 30, 2020, that the mechanism to import medicine to Iran without any glitches had been activated. This commercial channel for exporting medicine to Iran started processing its first payments on a pilot basis on January 27. It is said it would be fully operational in the immediate future. On February 2, the Swiss Embassy in Tehran tweeted: "Today, some 180,000 packs of transplant medication — part of the pilot transaction of the Swiss Humanitarian Trade Arrangement (SHTA) — have arrived at Tehran IKA airport. Thanks to a strong due diligence mechanism, the SHTA will ensure that products reach Iranian patients."[12]

Swiss Embassy Iran
@SwissEmbassyIr

Today, some 180'000 packs of transplant medication - part of the pilot transaction of the Swiss Humanitarian Trade Arrangement (SHTA) - have arrived at Tehran IKA airport. Thanks to a strong due diligence mechanism, the SHTA will ensure that products reach Iranian patients.

6:59 AM · Feb 2, 2020 · Twitter Web App

In reaction to dispatch of Swiss medicine to Iran, Abdolnaser Hemmati, the Governor of Iran's Central Bank said on February 3, "The amount of foreign currency that has been provided by the Central Bank for medicine and medical equipment and has been imported to Iran in the past ten months is over four billion dollars... Because of the endeavors of the Central Bank and other government institutions, we have pushed back sanctions, and the necessary medicines have been provided. The trend will continue in the future."[13]

Palpably, Abbas Mousavi, the Foreign Ministry Spokesman, said on February 4, "We do not recognize humanitarian channels or anything similar. We do not

---

12   Swiss Embassy Iran. Twitter Post. February 2, 2020, 6:59 A.M. https://twitter.com/SwissEmbassyIr/status/1223939038341730304

13   (Arman State-Run Newspaper, December 19, 2019), https://bit.ly/39IwYwS

recognize the sanctions. Medicine and food were not sanctioned, so no channel was needed to provide them and to create all this ballyhoo."[14]

In a press release discussing "Khamenei's lies" on March 23, Secretary of State Mike Pompeo said: "U.S. sanctions do not target imports of food, medicine and medical equipment, or other humanitarian goods. Iranian documents show their health companies have been able to import testing kits without obstacle from U.S. sanctions since January. The United States has offered over $100 million in medical assistance to foreign countries, including to the Iranian people. … Khamenei rejected this offer because he works tirelessly to concoct conspiracy theories and prioritizes ideology over the Iranian people."[15]

Another fact sheet entitled "Iran's Sanctions Relief Scam," released by the U.S. Department of State on April 6, 2020, accurately states that Iranian regime's "slick foreign influence campaign to obtain sanctions relief is not intended for the relief or health of the Iranian people but to raise funds for its terror operations. Since 2012, the regime has spent over $16 billion to fund its terror proxies abroad while Iranian healthcare services have remained woefully underfunded. This led the Iranian Health Minister to resign in January 2019 in protest of repeated health budget cuts."[16]

The regime's official news agency, IRNA, quoted the director-general of the World Health Organization on March 19: "Tedros Adhanom, head of WHO, said in response to a question about the organization's role in requesting a reduction of the impact of US sanctions against Iran during the current medical period and the spread of coronavirus, that he spoke on the phone with the US Secretary of State in this regard and that he emphasized the need to support Iran as it fights coronavirus. The director-general of WHO added: 'The US has agreed to suspend some of the sanctions against Iran, particularly in the realm of banking, in urgent circumstances and emergencies.'"[17]

---

14   "Az News TV," Aznews TV, February 3, 2020, https://www.aznews.tv/

15   Michael Pompeo, "Khamenei's Lies About the Wuhan Virus Put Lives at Risk — United States Department of State," U.S. Department of State (U.S. Department of State, February 23, 2020), https://www.state.gov/khameneis-lies-about-the-wuhan-virus-put-lives-at-risk/

16   "Iran's Sanctions Relief Scam," U.S. Department of State, April 6, 2020, https://www.state.gov/irans-sanctions-relief-scam/

17   KhabarFori, April 5, 2020, https://www.khabarfoori.com/detail/1756982

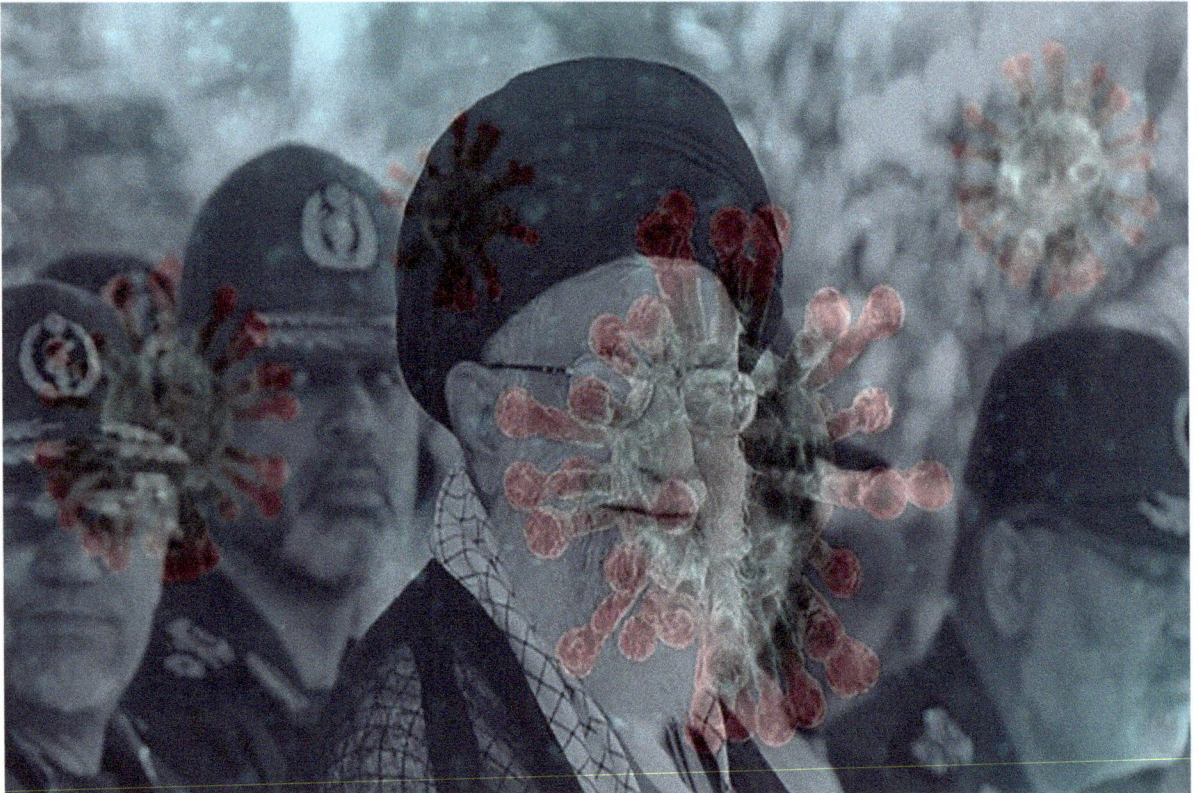

Clearly, for Khamenei and his regime, including the whitewashed image of Tehran offered by the Zarif foreign ministry, the issue is not the pain and suffering of the Iranian people. Rather, they are trying to exploit the fatal coronavirus disaster to their own advantage, hoping to reduce the regime's international isolation and sanctions.

There is a long-standing pattern of opportunism in the regime's policies placing the interests of the corrupt religious dictatorship ahead of the lives of Iran's citizens. At the start of the regime's rule, Khomeini described the war between Iran and Iraq, which sent hundreds and perhaps thousands of people to their deaths on a daily basis, as a "divine gift." He sought in the midst of war and slaughter to erect the foundations of his regime. Today, Khomeini's followers view the coronavirus in the same light, not as a threat to the lives of innocent civilians, but as an "opportunity" for their regime to free themselves of sanctions by leveraging the crisis.

Terrorism Overrides Healthcare

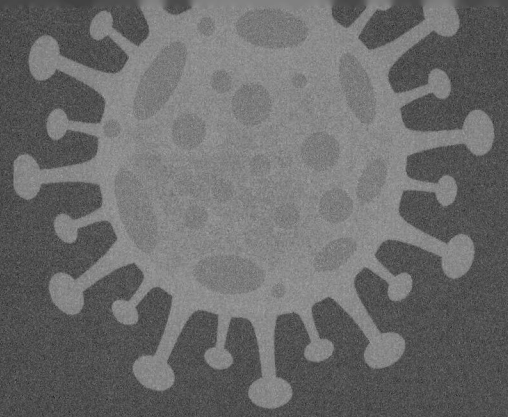

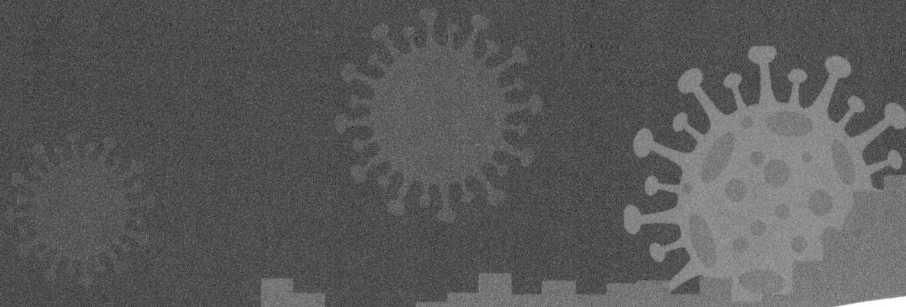

A review of the state budget announced by Rouhani for the Persian calendar year 1397 (March 2018 to March 2019) , which was delivered to parliament in December 2017, shows that the total budget was $121.5B.[18] Out of this amount, $26.8B, or 22%, was allocated to military and security affairs and export of fundamentalism. In addition, institutions controlled by Supreme Leader Khamenei and the IRGC dedicate an unofficial budget to military, security and fundamentalism affairs, which for that year equaled $27.5B. That brings the total amount dedicated to the regime's domestic suppression, foreign adventurism and terrorism outside its borders to about $55B.

In the 2018 budget, only $16.3B was allocated to healthcare for 80 million Iranians. In other words, Iranians pay three times the amount spent on the country's healthcare for the dictatorship's repression and spread of global terrorism.

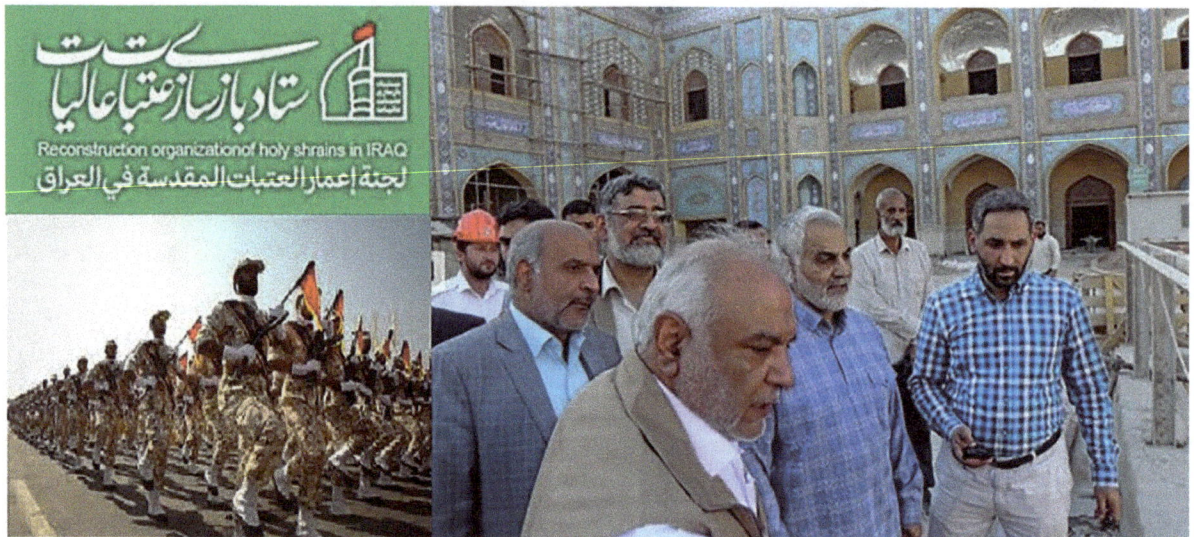

The deceased IRGC Qods Force commander, Qassem Soleimani seen with leaders of Iraqi Shiite militias visiting one of the religious centers where the Iranian regime spent a large sum of money. In fact, the regime in Tehran has set up what it calls "Reconstruction Organization of Holy Shrines in Iraq."

---

18   Calculated using an exchange rate of 3,500 Tomans, which was accounted for by the budget bill itself.

Theft and Hoarding of Medical Resources

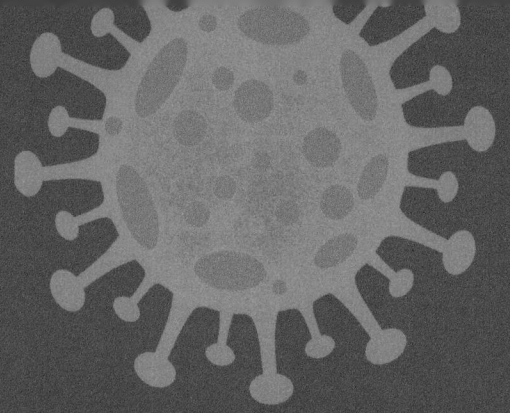

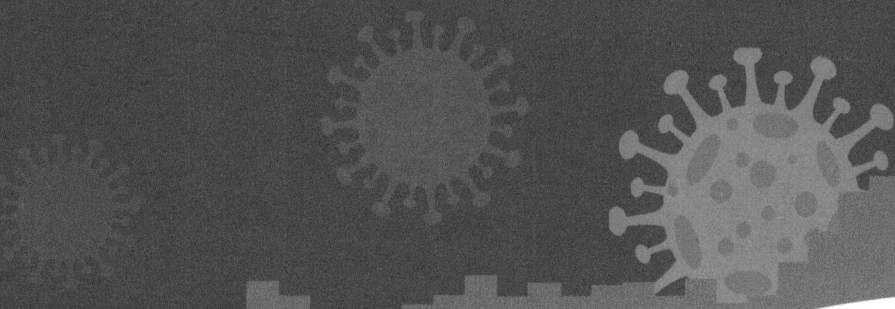

Regime officials falsely claim that the spread of coronavirus in Iran and the high death toll are caused by the lack of medical resources stemming from sanctions. This much is clear, even from officials' own statements: the coronavirus pandemic has become yet another source of plunder by the regime's corrupt factions and the IRGC. The resources provided to Iran to counter the virus are not going to the Iranian people; instead they enter the black market, which in turn creates shortages and causes more deaths.

State-affiliated entities hid medical masks in warehouses during the first days of the coronavirus outbreak and sold them on the black market to poverty-stricken and desperate people at five times the normal price. The regime also sent as gifts five million masks to China and two million masks to its proxies in Iraq in an attempt to advance its own policies in the region and relevant to China.

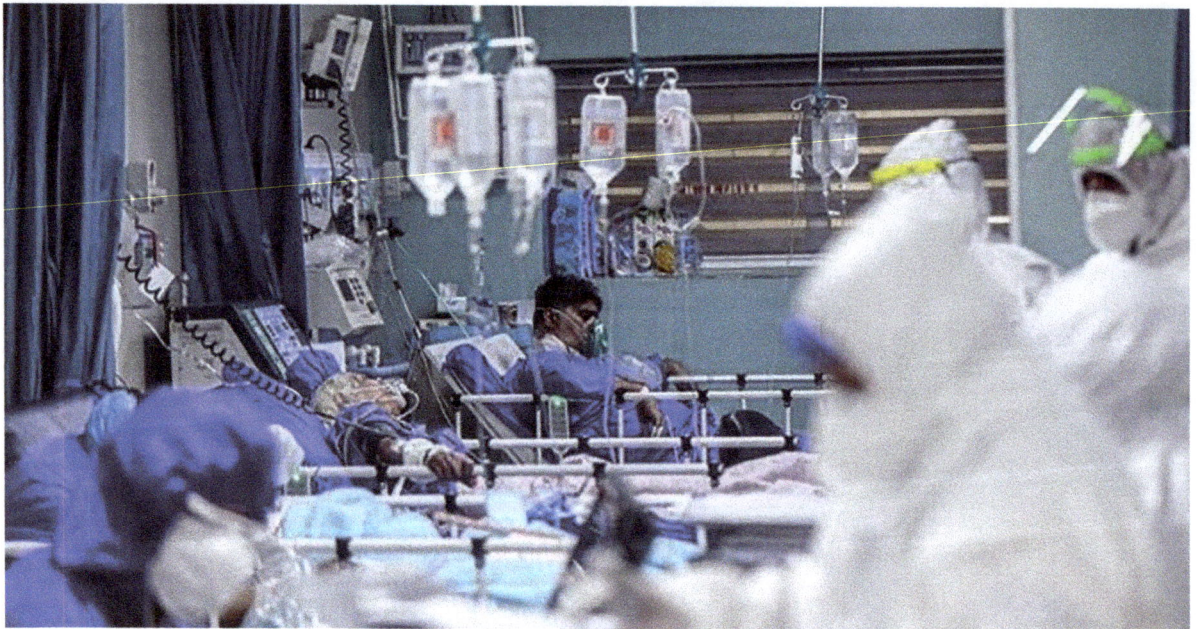

The state-run website Qods Online reported on July 20, 2019, that at least one billion euros from the state's foreign reserve account had been lost. "Mahmoud Vaezi, the president's Chief of Staff, has asked four ministers in a letter to provide explanations about 'commitments made in terms of foreign currency allocations (totaling about one billion euros) which have not been respected for the import of medicine and other necessary products.'"[19]

---

19   Quds Online News-Analytical website, (July 20, 2019), http://bit.ly/2LtEdRv

Another state-run website, Fararu, also published a report about corruption in the Health Ministry, focusing on an astronomical embezzlement. The report says: "The most recent case of corruption that has been disclosed concerns the disappearance of $1.3B in foreign currency obtained at 4,200 Tomans in order to import medical equipment. It is not clear what this money was spent on and which non-medical purposes it was used for."[20]

According to this report, Health Minister Saeid Namaki reacted to the organized corruption in the fields of medicine and medical equipment, writing on his Instagram page: "$1.3B of foreign currency for medical equipment is gone and it is not precisely clear yet who has taken this money and what they have obtained for it and whom they have given it to." He added: "We are dealing with organized corruption in the fields of medicine and medical equipment, involving even some

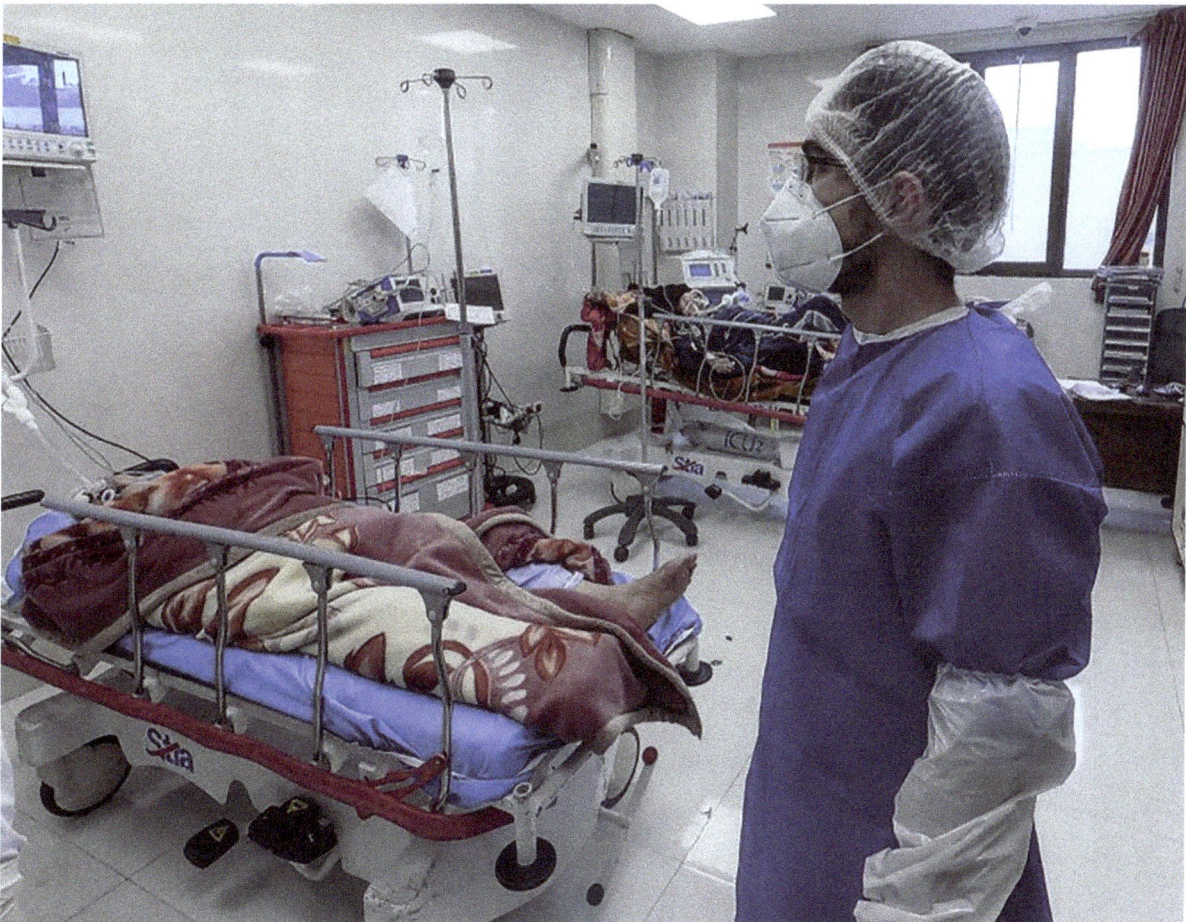

---

20   Fararu, July 20, 2019, https://bit.ly/2wbZiK6

companies with ties to the Health Ministry. I am not afraid to say that many of these companies that have ties to the board of directors providing foreign currency are problematic (corrupt) in one way or another."

After the spread of coronavirus in Iran, Namaki wrote a letter to the regime's Supreme National Security Council, regarding the state-run smugglers and mafia network that hoard preventative medical equipment for treatment of coronavirus: "I predicted the probability of the coronavirus coming into the country in a letter to the country's customs and requested that the export of masks be prohibited until further notice. I instructed my colleagues to purchase domestic products at a rational price and store them for the worst-case scenario. Unfortunately, despite many follow-ups, a small number were purchased and the rest of the country's products entered the black market. Unfortunately, after about 10 days, only a million masks were provided and I do not know where the rest have been stored. My colleagues are forced to work on a daily basis searching various markets and playing the role of middlemen to purchase these products at astronomical prices from smugglers.[21]

"My question is ... during a period when there is a probability of people being infected as a result of a lack of protective and preventive equipment, on what basis does this opportunistic and unreasonable network dare to stand up to the people and officials and simply declare that it can provide 200,000,000 masks in the span of 24 hours in this or that market at this or that price? Is it fair that a group of people sacrifice their lives to protect the people while another group hoard the first group's protective gear and masks, as well as those that belong to patients, in order to profit hundreds of times over or to smuggle these items to other countries?"[22]

Namaki said in another letter to the Minister of Mines and Industries, Reza Rahmani, who had claimed that his ministry is producing millions of masks and other products: "Saying that several million masks are being produced on a daily basis is misleading the public. We have obtained one million masks so far. ... Unfortunately, we are still grappling with the lack of masks, and according to

---

21   Tasnim News Agency, March 1, 2020, https://bit.ly/34aT4XD

22   Fars News Agency, February 29, 2020, https://bit.ly/2V9GKma

information obtained, a convoluted network of hoarders is selling masks at 10 times the regular price."[23]

It is abundantly clear that Namaki's reference to the "network" is actually the state mafia affiliated with the IRGC and the State Security Forces (SSF). There are no private entities that can "provide 200,000,000 masks in the span of 24 hours in this or that market at this or that price."

Another instance involves the fraudulent sale of air fresheners packaged as anti-bacterial sprays. These items are produced at IRGC factories and sold to ordinary people at several times the average price. Similarly, sanitizer solutions gifted from Germany are sold on the black market at about $18 a bottle (75,000 Tomans).

To hide the reality and prevent the regime from being blamed, officials claim that the theft and hoarding of medicine is the work of ordinary businessmen and the public. However, there are absolutely no entities that have no state ties and are involved in hoarding and smuggling on this vast scale.

23   Ebtekar Newspaper, accessed April 4, 2020, https://bit.ly/39IGGz1

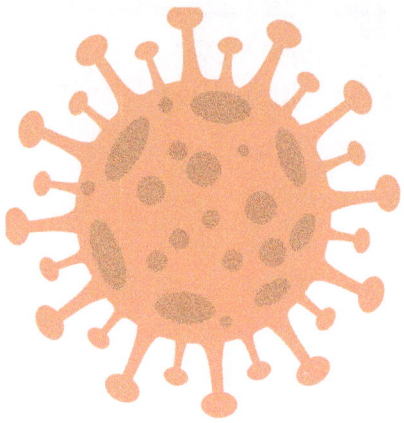

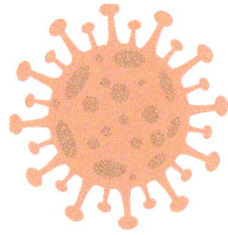

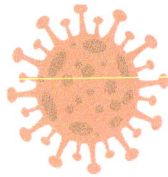

The Iranian People's Wealth in the Hands of Khamenei and the IRGC

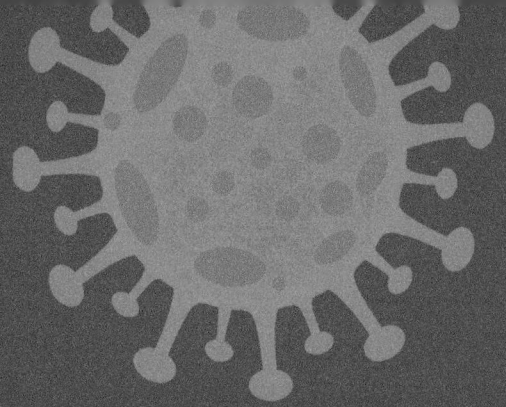

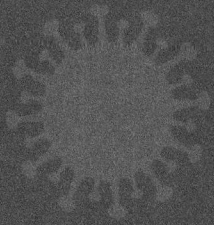

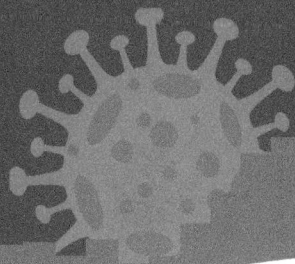

All over the world, governments are going out of their way to alleviate the suffering of the people in combating the coronavirus. Iran is the one country where the regime and the people are on two different sides. The regime's efforts are aimed at covering up the actual figures and dealing with political consequences, namely thwarting any expression of public outrage in response to its mismanagement of the virus. This has contributed significantly to people's dire predicament and hardships.

While Khamenei has refused using his personal coffer to provide for the most basic needs of Iranians, the salary and benefits of repressive forces namely the IRGC and the regime's proxies outside are continuing to be paid. On January 8, the regime increased the budget of the IRGC Qods Force by 200 million Euros.

REUTERS INVESTIGATES   *About the series* ⓘ

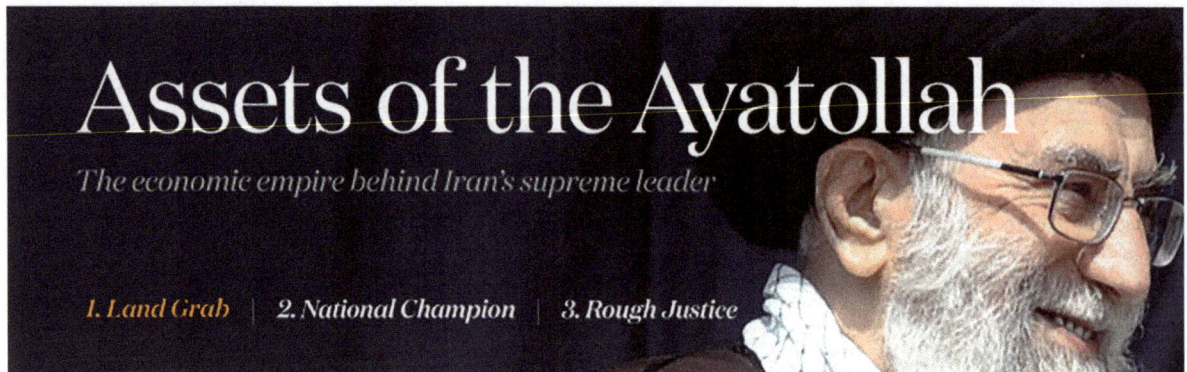

Assets of the Ayatollah
The economic empire behind Iran's supreme leader

1. Land Grab | *2. National Champion* | *3. Rough Justice*

Khamenei controls massive financial empire built on property seizures

Behzad Nabavi, a former government spokesman and former deputy speaker of the regime's parliament, has said: "60% of Iran's wealth is in the hands of four entities: the Setad-e Ejraee Farman-e Imam, Khatam Base, Astan-e Qods, and the Mostazafan Foundation."[24]

---

24   "Four Khamenei-Linked Institutions Own 60% Of Iran's National Assets, Says Politician," RFE/RL (Iran News By Radio Farda, September 22, 2019), https://en.radiofarda.com/a/four-khamenei-linked-institutions-own-60-percent-of-iran-s-national-assets-says-politician/30177579.html

Of these four entities, three are directly supervised by the regime's Supreme Leader, Ali Khamenei. The fourth, the Khatam al-Anbiya Garrison, is affiliated with the IRGC, which itself is under the direct control of Khamenei.

The state-run daily Ebtekar said on March 9, 2020: The chairman and three members of the Citizens' Rights faction in parliament demanded an order be issued by the Supreme National Security Council to place crisis centers under 100% quarantine. Abdolkarim Hosseinzadeh, Tayyebeh Siavoshi, Fatemeh Saeedi, and Seyyedeh Hamideh Zarabadi, wrote on their personal accounts on Twitter: "Preventing the spread of coronavirus has not been successful for whatever reason. Two necessary steps: 1 — An order by the Supreme National Security Council to place crisis centers under 100% quarantine. 2 — Use the replete resources of the Social Security Investment Company, the Setad-e Imam, the Mostazafan Foundation and Petrochemical holdings to procure and distribute masks, suits, glasses and other necessary medical supplies."[25]

Hence, it is clear even in the eyes of the regime's own officials where the Iranian people's money has been stored and out of which accounts the necessary costs for the prevention and countering of coronavirus must be spent. These entities have tens of billions of dollars in assets and cash on hand. Additionally, one of the biggest institutions that is tied to the regime and which spends its money only on the authority of Khamenei is the National Development Fund. Currently, it has a reserve worth tens of billions of dollars.

These institutions are tax-exempt. Their annual balance sheets and cash flow statements are not published and no one can hold them accountable. Their activities are confidential and reports about their conduct are rarely publicized in the media. Obtaining information about their contracts and net worth is extremely difficult.

The Social Security Investment Company is another enormous cartel for plunder used by rival factions. It holds billions of dollars and has an annual net return of one billion dollars.

---

25   Twitter Post. March 8, 2020, 7:30 A.M.
      https://twitter.com/H_Zarabadi/status/1236615152583270401

Providing detailed descriptions of these economic powerhouses requires pages of documentation. Only a brief treatment follows. (For more information on these entities please see Appendix II).

"SETAD"

"SETAD" refers to the Headquarters for Executing the Order of the Imam.[26] A Reuters investigation published on November 11, 2013, which was the result of a six-month investigation, estimated its assets at about $95 billion. According to Reuters, the $95B figure comes from analyzing official statements by SETAD authorities, figures obtained from the Tehran stock exchange, company websites, and information from the US Treasury.

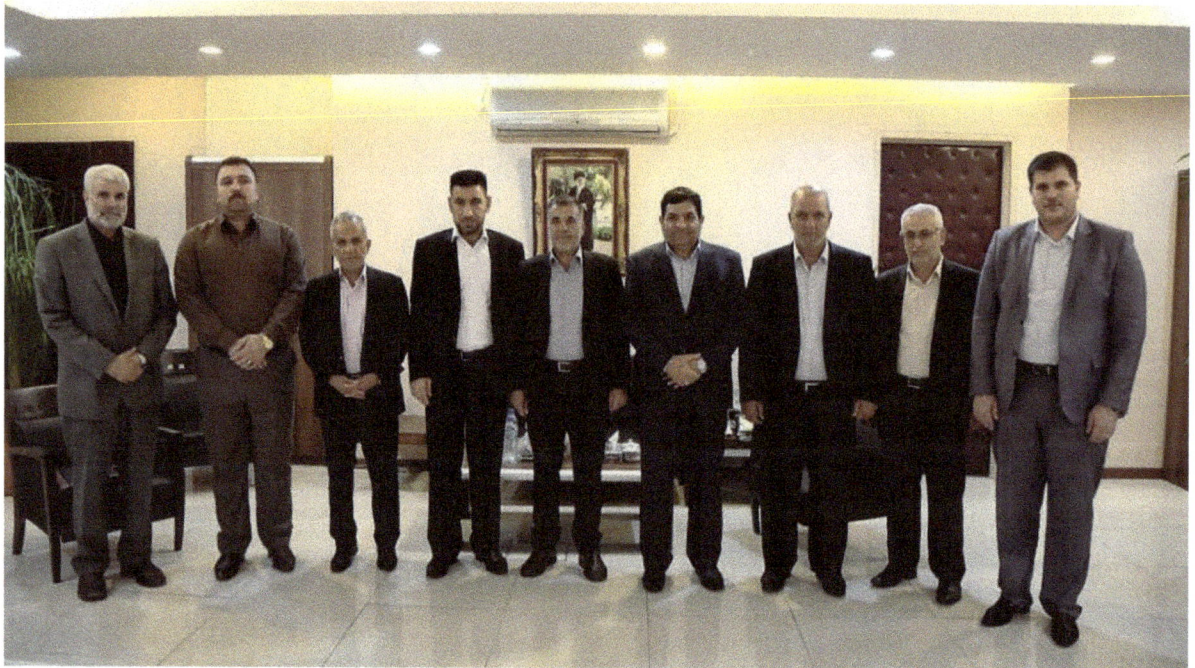

Leaders of Iraqi Shiite militia meet the head of SETAD which funds their terror operations in Iraq.

---

26 *Iran: The Rise of the Revolutionary Guards Financial Empire: How the Supreme Leader and IRGC Rob the People to Fund International Terror* (Washington, D. C.: National Council of Resistance of Iran, 2017) , p.76

Astan-e Qods Razavi

Astan-e Qods Razavi is the largest endowment institution in the Islamic world.[27] The organization and management of all the religious ceremonies and financial gifts for the shrine of the eighth Shiite Imam over the past several centuries have been controlled by the Astan-e Qods, whose head is directly appointed by the Supreme Leader. Over the past 42 years, three people have been handpicked by Khamenei to run this vast institution: Mullah Abbas Vaez Tabasi who died in March 2016; Ebrahim Raisi, current head of Khamenei's Judiciary and member of the death commission during the 1988 massacre in Iran; and mullah Ahmad Marvi, a close Khamenei confidant. No one other than Khamenei himself has the authority to hold this economic powerhouse accountable.

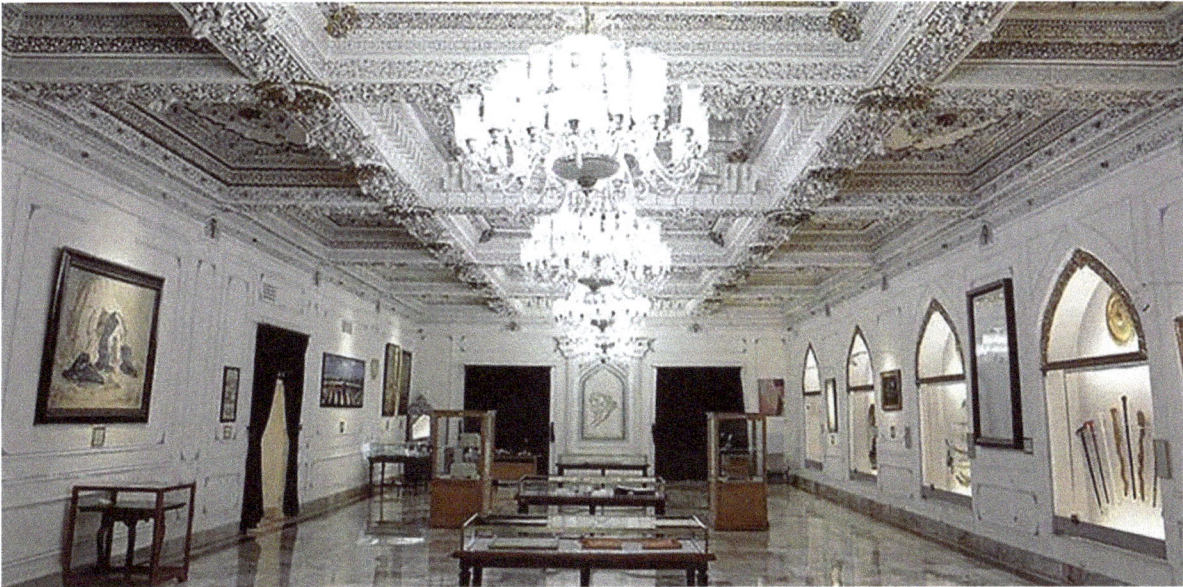

One of the museums of the Astan-e Qods Razavi

---

27   *Ibid*, p.84

The Mostazafan Foundation

The Mostazafan Foundation is controlled by the Supreme Leader and governed through a board of directors. The foundation oversees close to 140 companies in the food, chemical, petrochemical, metals, building, agricultural and tourism industries. Owing to its special legal status, it can work directly with foreign companies.[28]

In the past, the Mostazafan Foundation was considered the largest economic powerhouse in Iran. Today, it has over 200,000 employees.[29]

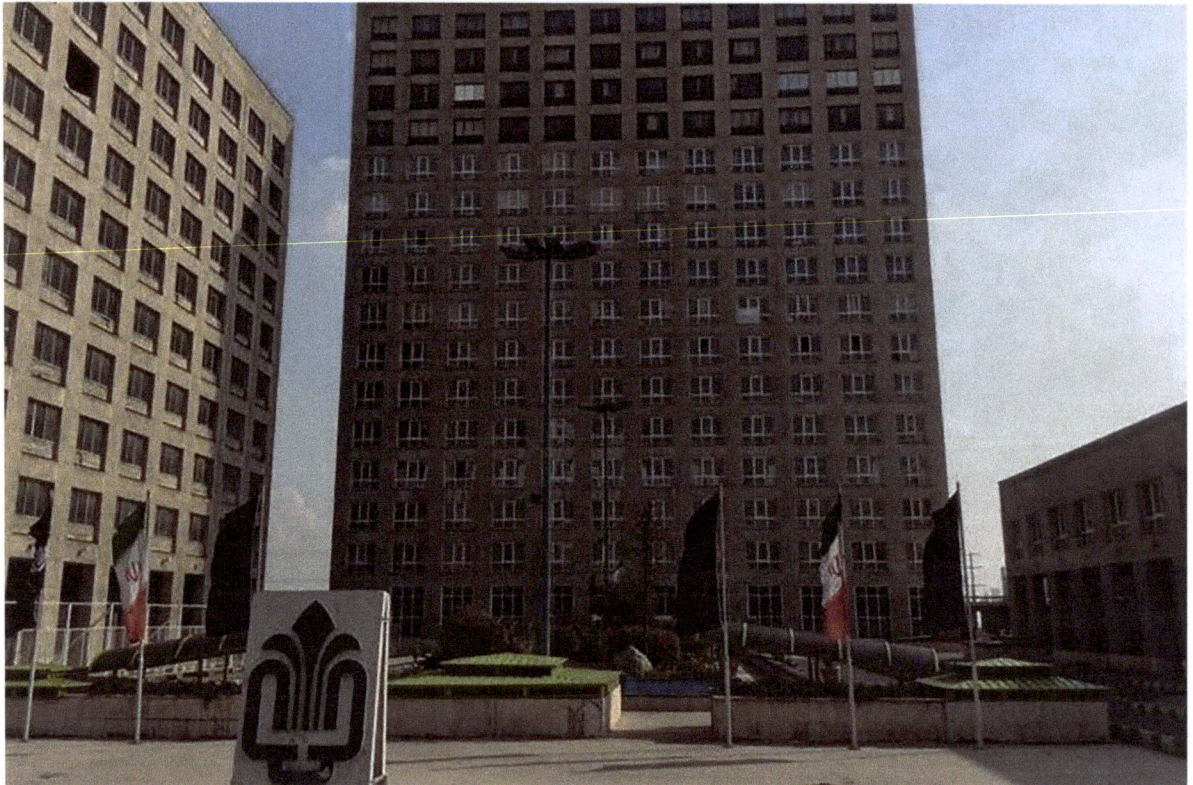

The headquarters of the Mostazafan Foundation in Tehran

---

28 In 1989, Mostazafan Foundation controlled over 800 companies and commercial entities, all of which were confiscated properties. After the so-called privatization and transfer of state assets to private entities, the number of these companies was reduced to 400 in 1999.

29 *Iran: The Rise of the Revolutionary Guards Financial Empire*, p.81

Khatam al-Anbiya Construction Headquarters

The Khatam al-Anbiya Construction Headquarters is the main financial and commercial arm of the Islamic Revolutionary Guard Corps (IRGC). It began its activities as a contractor of industrial and construction projects following the ceasefire in the Iran-Iraq War in 1989. Khatam is the largest contractor for government projects in Iran. It has 5,000 subcontractors and about 135,000 employees.[30]

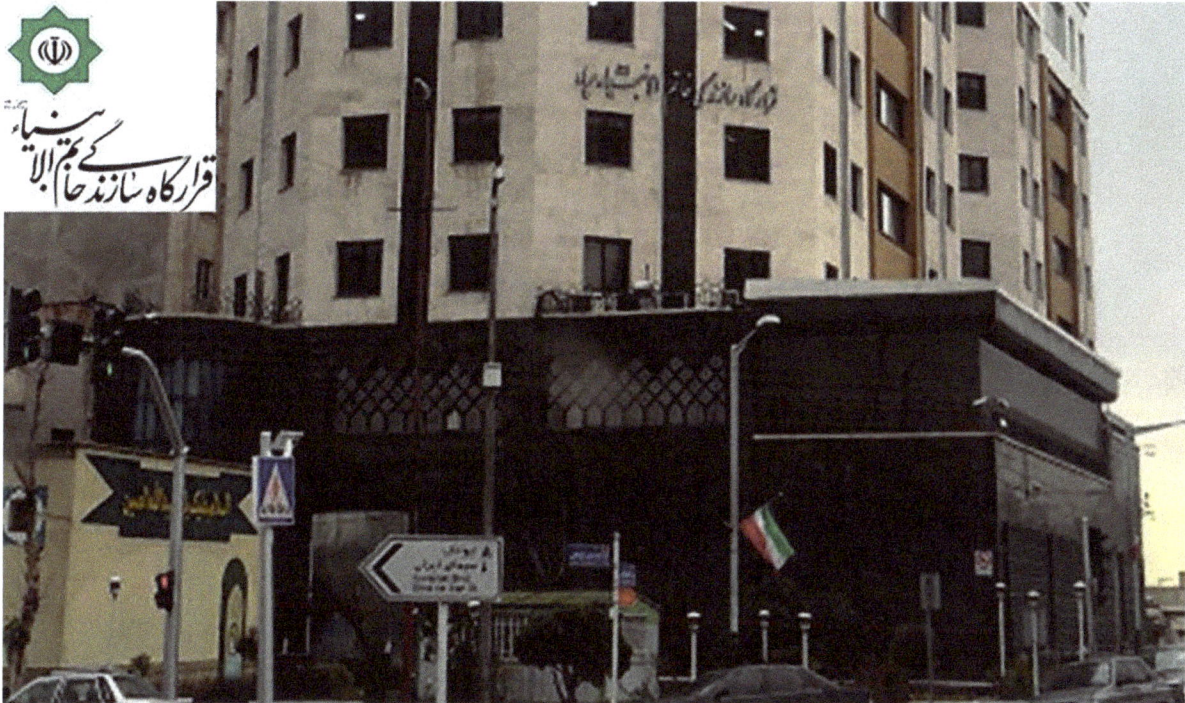

One of the offices of the Khatam al-Anbiya Construction Headquarters

---

30 IRGC Brig. Gen. Abadollah Abdollahi, then-commander of Khatam al-Anbiya, state-run Sharq Daily, December 17, 2014

Social Security Investment Company

The Social Security Investment Company is a holding company and was established by the Social Security Organization as a special investment arm with an initial capital of close to $500,000. The company is active in investments, commerce, trade, management and investment banking. Six years ago, close to 10% of all the value of the Tehran Stock Exchange belonged to the company's subsidiaries.[31]

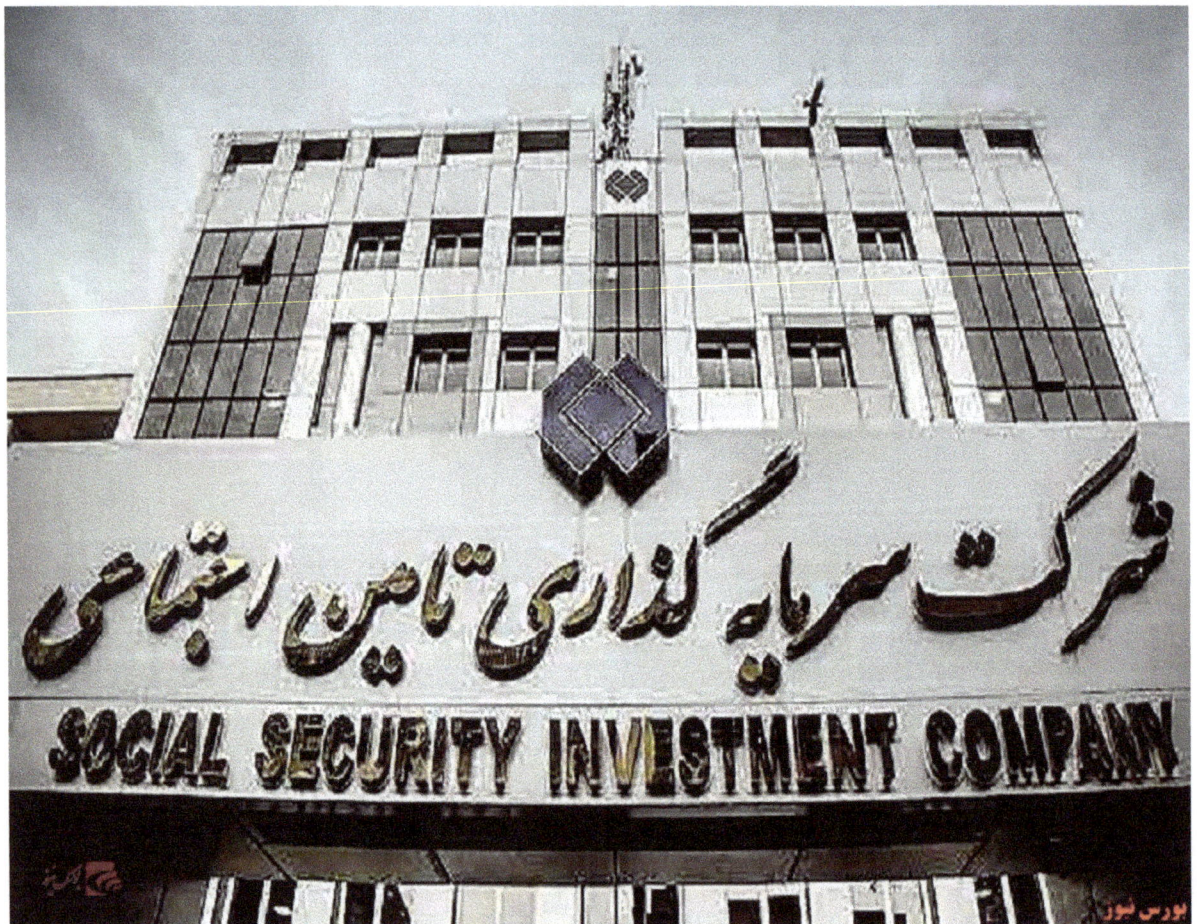

---

31   Alef News Site, August 2, 2014, accessed April 4, 2020, https://bit.ly/3bXIoym

The National Development Fund

Another monetary source for the clerical regime worth tens of billions of dollars is the National Development Fund. This fund was set up to invest in the regime's long-term economic projects, but the authority over its spending rests with Supreme Leader Khamenei. The latest report on the fund came out on March 26, 2020, when urgent medical needs were expressed.

Since the coronavirus epidemic in Iran, some of the regime's officials have pointed to the reserves in the National Development Fund to address medical needs.[32]

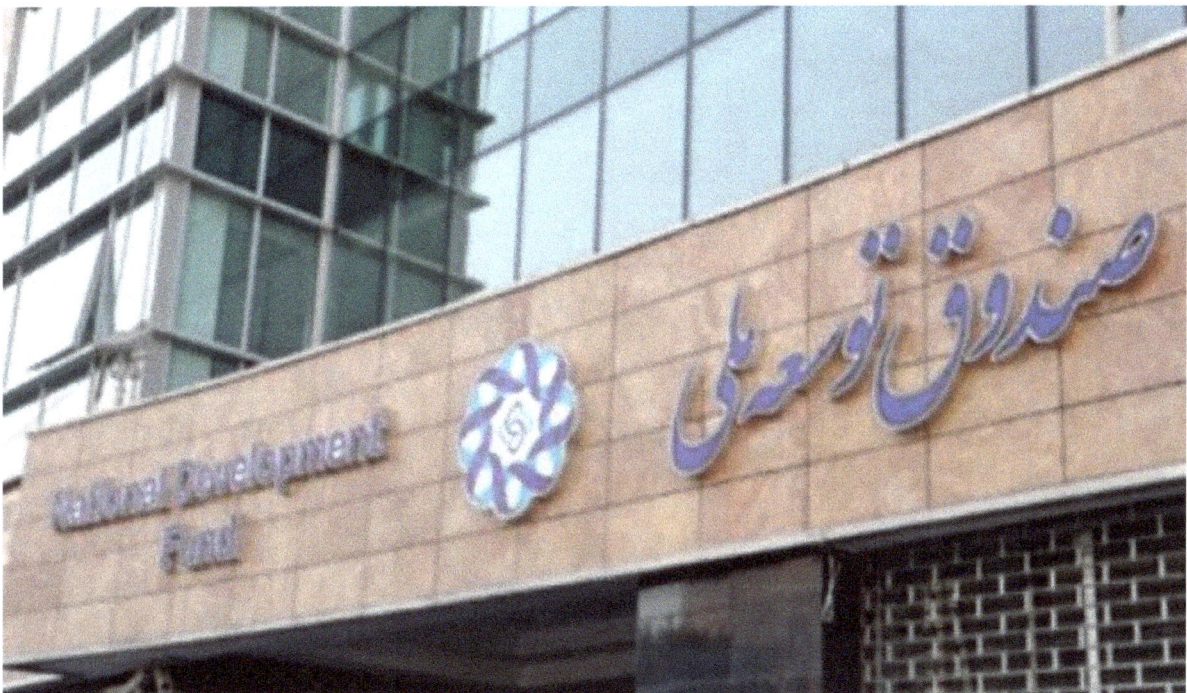

---

32   Etemad Online, March 7, 2020, accessed April 5, 2020, https://bit.ly/34acj3o

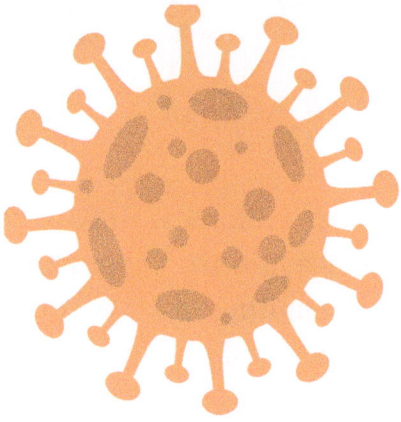

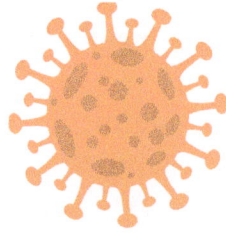

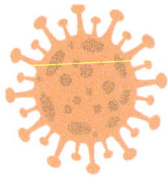

Khamenei and Rouhani Sending People Back to Work at the Height of the Pandemic

On April 5, in a meeting with the coronavirus task force, the regime's president, Hassan Rouhani, urged government employees as well as others to go back to work. Rouhani set April 11 as the start date for low risk "businesses," and "economic activities." He said, "We are using a step-by-step process to reopen services... Starting from next week, government agencies will start working with two-thirds of their employees; a third will be allowed to stay at home."

Rouhani brazenly declared: "We have white (virus-free) provinces in the south of the country, where there are no problems for schools to open. Bushehr, Hormozgan, Sistan & Baluchestan Provinces ... can start their activities." His statement sharply contradicted what the spokesman for the regime's Health Ministry said on the same day: "No provinces are considered white as it relates to the coronavirus outbreak."

During the same week, the Health Minister, Healthcare Organization, and many other regime officials had warned against resuming administrative and financial activities. The Health Minister warned that any such decision would impact "the health of the people and then the economy." He pleaded, "Please don't be careless; we are still in the process of managing the disease, not containing and controlling the patients."

On April 4th, Seyed Hassan Inanlou, deputy director of treatment at Alborz University of Medical Sciences, warned that if people pursue their ordinary lives due to financial reasons, "the disease will explode, hospitals will be overloaded with patients, we will lose control, and won't be able to manage the outbreak." He suggested that "a million people will die."

The criminal decision by the regime's Supreme Leader, Khamenei, and his president to order the people back to work will endanger the health of millions of Iranians. Instead of providing the minimum means of subsistence to the Iranian people from the funds in economic entities controlled by Khamenei and the IRGC, which have been stolen from the Iranian nation in the first place, the mullahs' regime is sending the Iranian people to the altar of coronavirus. Incompetence, pilfering, political considerations, and tremendous class differences under the ruling theocracy aggravate the scope of the catastrophe. The regime fears that economic pressure might lead to a mass uprising and undermine its survival.

Attacking Americans in Iraq to Divert Attention Away from the Coronavirus Crisis

In recent weeks, attacks by the regime's proxy forces against the bases housing American forces in Iraq have increased substantially. Baghdad's Green Zone and the area housing the American embassy in Iraq have been targeted. According to al-Hurra TV, the attack on Taji base on March 12, 2020 marked the 22nd attack since January by regime forces against American targets.[33] The March 12 assault against coalition forces in northern Baghdad was unprecedented in recent years. It involved the firing of 18 Katyusha rockets, leaving two American soldiers and one British soldier dead and 10 others wounded. Sky News Arabic on March 12 quoted an American analyst as saying: "In reality, there are only two parties that attack US forces in Iraq: the Iranian regime and the Hashd al-Shaabi. It is inconceivable for anyone to believe that these are not one entity. This is not only a fact, but it is also the official stance of the US government. It is amazing that this attack against Taji was repeated two days later on March 14, which led to only the wounding of several people."[34] *The Washington Examiner* wrote: "Both attacks were carried out by Iran's Kata'ib Hezbollah militia proxy, under direction from Iran's IRGC. But what makes these attacks particularly concerning is that they are designed to kill."[35]

No one doubts that Kata'ib Hezbollah is actually a branch of the Qods Force that is operating inside Iraq, especially in light of the fact that the attack took place two days after the visit of IRGC general Ali Shamkhani, who is also the Secretary General of the regime's Supreme National Security Council and Khamenei's special envoy to Iraq. Shamkhani wrote in his twitter account: "It seems like there are commonalities between the assassination (of Soleimani and associates) and the US claim about attacks on the Taji base in Baghdad."

Removing all doubt about who is responsible for the attack on Taji, the website Iranian Diplomacy, which is run by Sadeq Kharrazi, a former regime ambassador to France and a close friend of Soleimani and Zarif, referred to the military and political background of Shamkhani and wrote: "All this makes him the best

---

33   Anadolu Agency, March 14, 2020, accessed April 4, 2020, https://bit.ly/3aTw3KP

34   Anadolu Agency, March 14, 2020, accessed April 4, 2020, https://bit.ly/3aTw3KP

35   Tom Rogan, "The US May Have to Target the IRGC in Iran to Stop Iraq Base Attacks," Washington Examiner, March 15, 2020, https://www.washingtonexaminer.com/opinion/the-us-may-have-to-target-the-irgc-in-iran-to-stop-iraq-base-attacks

alternative to replace Soleimani in order to manage the Iraqi affairs."[36] Although Esmail Qaani has replaced Soleimani as the Qods Force commander, intelligence from inside the regime also indicates that the void in Iraq will be filled by Shamkhani.

In view of the fact that the launch of every missile has to be approved by Khamenei himself, as announced by the Chairman of the Joint Chiefs of Staff of the regime's Armed Forces, Hassan Firouzabadi, why has the regime resorted to such acts? The answer can best be traced to the ongoing coronavirus crisis inside Iran. It is clear that the regime is mired in this domestic crisis, which can and likely will define the end for the dictatorship. The regime knows full well that the Iranian people are extremely angry over its corruption, mismanagement, hoarding and theft of medical equipment. This rage will explode as the coronavirus crisis expands beyond the control of the regime. For self-protection, the regime needs to create another crisis — a foreign crisis — to divert attention away from the internal coronavirus pandemic.

In view of the fact that the US government is grappling with the same crisis, as well as the presidential election campaign, the regime likely calculates that the Trump administration will be reluctant to act forcefully. Hence the regime feels safe to exploit the situation, attacking Americans and crossing red lines.

Whatever the calculations, it is clear that the clerical regime is not willing to retreat in any way from its inhumane behavior toward the Iranian people or its regional aggression. The regime has no flexibility. On the contrary, it will involve itself in more killings, terrorism, foreign adventurism and other crimes. The only language that the regime respects is the language of force.

---

36   Iranian Diplomacy, March 11, 2020, accessed April 4, 2020, https://bit.ly/2xQUw5t

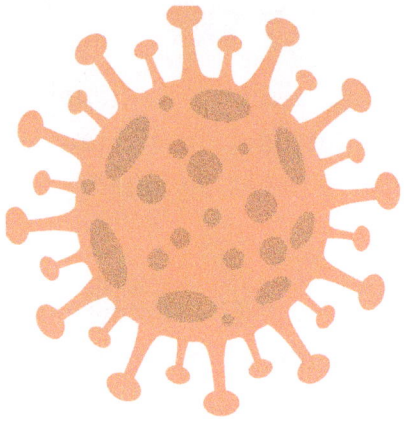

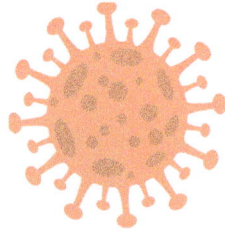

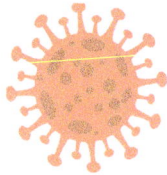

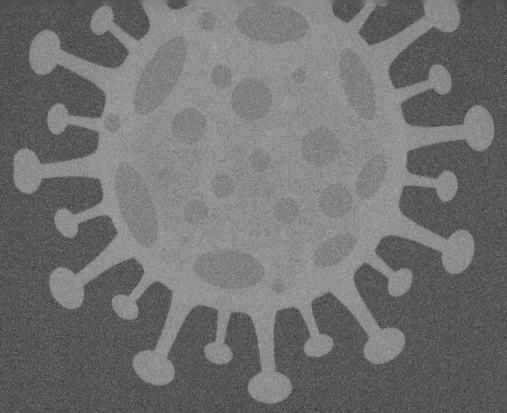

Conclusion

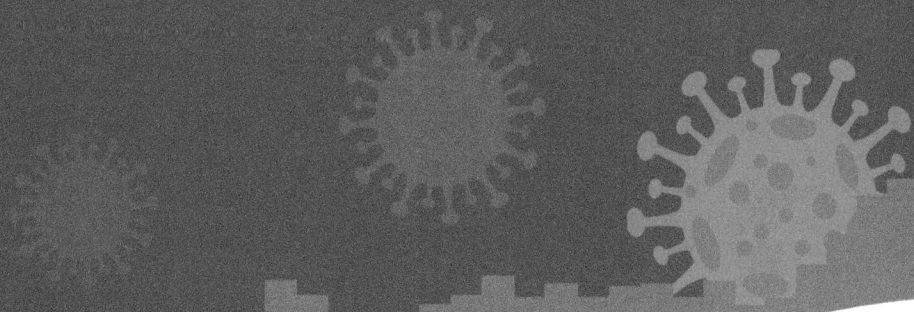

The Iran regime pursues a two-pronged strategy in dealing with the coronavirus crisis. At home, it tries to cover up the number of fatalities and its failure, prompted by political and economic considerations, to adopt the measures needed to prevent the spread of the virus. At the international level, its talking heads, lobbyists and appeasement advocates claim that the sanctions are hampering its efforts to effectively manage the crisis. The mullahs' duplicity and attempts to conceal their ulterior motives and incompetence, are undermined by the facts on the ground, which demonstrate that the regime, and only the regime, is responsible for the disastrous spread of the epidemic, resulting in the shocking death toll.

Crocodile tears do nothing for the Iranian people; practical and immediate steps are needed to help them, and those steps do not include throwing a lifeline to the moribund ruling regime. The mullahs must be compelled to allow international organizations into Iran to provide direct help. In lieu of spending vast sums on the IRGC's Quds Force or its terrorist proxies outside Iran, the regime must be forced to allocate the nation's wealth to the task of confronting the coronavirus.

Iran's theocracy has no regard for the people's health and well-being. This was evident in November 2019, when it murdered over 1,500 protesters demanding their basic freedoms. In January 2020, the regime shot down a passenger plane, killing all on board, and lied about it for days. Afterwards, it went after the families of the victims who demanded accountability and justice for their loved ones. It has yet to provide the plane's black box for international examination, or to prosecute anyone for this crime.

That level of cold-blooded criminal indifference has again been evident during the coronavirus crisis, in which the regime not only played a critical role, but also deliberately covered up, causing the virus to spread like wildfire to all 31 provinces. There is reliable evidence that the regime knew about the impending crisis as early as late January, but did not inform the public or the world in order to ensure a higher turnout for the revolution anniversary march on February 11 and the sham parliamentary elections on February 21. The IRGC-controlled Mahan Air continued passenger flights to and from China well into March. Several hundred

Chinese clerics were allowed to study in Qom, where the virus was first detected and from where it spread to other Iranian provinces.

Abdolreza Rahmani Fazli, the regime's Interior Minister, vehemently denied any coronavirus infection on February 1, 2020, saying, "Last night we held a meeting with the Minister of Health at the request of Vice President Eshaq Jahangiri to discuss the coronavirus. The Health Minister briefed us in detail, saying that we don't have any corona infection in Iran." Documents obtained by the People's Mojahedin Organization of Iran (PMOI/MEK) from the National Emergency Organization show that several coronavirus patients in Tehran had been hospitalized as early as January 2020.

Two days after the NCRI's Security and Counterterrorism Committee revealed on March 28 the first series of undeniable documents substantiating the presence of the coronavirus in Iran, Hassan Rouhani, in a startling retreat, said: "The disease may have been introduced as early as the third week of January 2020 in Iran, but we found out about it in the third week of February. It took us a while to know. All over the world it was like that! It took some time to realize they were facing the disease."

Tehran still refuses to provide accurate information about the number of fatalities. In late March, a World Health Organization official estimated that casualty figures could be five times higher than official reports suggest. The nearly month-long criminal cover-up was definitely a key factor in the rapid outbreak in Iran, a crime against humanity for which the regime's leaders must be brought to justice.

Meanwhile, corruption has reached cosmic proportions. Due to hoarding of supplies, price manipulation, and sheer mismanagement, hospitals lack basic necessities to confront the epidemic. The wealth of the Iranian nation must be used for the safety and health of its citizens. But it remains hidden in the institutions and foundations controlled by the Supreme Leader and the IRGC. The IRGC, for example, hoards and sells on the black-market basic items like masks and disinfectants at 10 times the average price. The Health Minister attested, "$1.3 billion dollars allotted to the purchase of medical supplies have gone missing."

While the rest of the world is fighting the coronavirus with social distancing, quarantine, and services and resources to the needy, so that they can stay home and save lives, the Iranian regime is doing the exact opposite. Rather than allocating the vast sums available to it to fund the fight against the crisis, it continues to fund terror groups in the region, escalating the threats against the Americans in Iraq and elsewhere.

As a state policy, the regime seeks to exploit the coronavirus and the loss of life to boost its own status by getting the sanctions lifted without abandoning the rogue behavior which caused the imposition of sanctions in the first place. Tehran is looking for cash to fund its terror operations in the region, while it rejects humanitarian and medical assistance by other nations, including the United States, as well as non-governmental organizations such as Doctors Without Borders.

As acknowledged by top regime officials, the mullahs do have the necessary means and resources to combat the coronavirus, but refrain from using them for the health and welfare of the Iranian people. Many bipartisan members of the U.S. Congress argue that there is no justification for lifting or easing sanctions, when the regime continues its support for terrorism, its missile and nuclear programs, and human rights violations at home.

The world community in general and the U.S. in particular can best help the victims of the coronavirus in Iran by taking the following steps:

1. Demand that the Iranian regime allow international humanitarian and medical assistance to be delivered directly to the people of Iran.

2. Force the Iranian regime to allocate the country's resources, including the billions which the Supreme Leader controls, to the fight against the coronavirus instead of allocating it to terror operations in the region.

3. The Iranian people have long considered Iran's repressive rulers as their main enemy. The Iranian regime's mishandling of the coronavirus crisis has further convinced them that the ultimate solution to bring freedom to Iran and stability to the Middle East is regime change. Europe and the United States

should recognize the right of the Iranian people to unseat the ayatollahs and establish freedom and democracy in Iran.

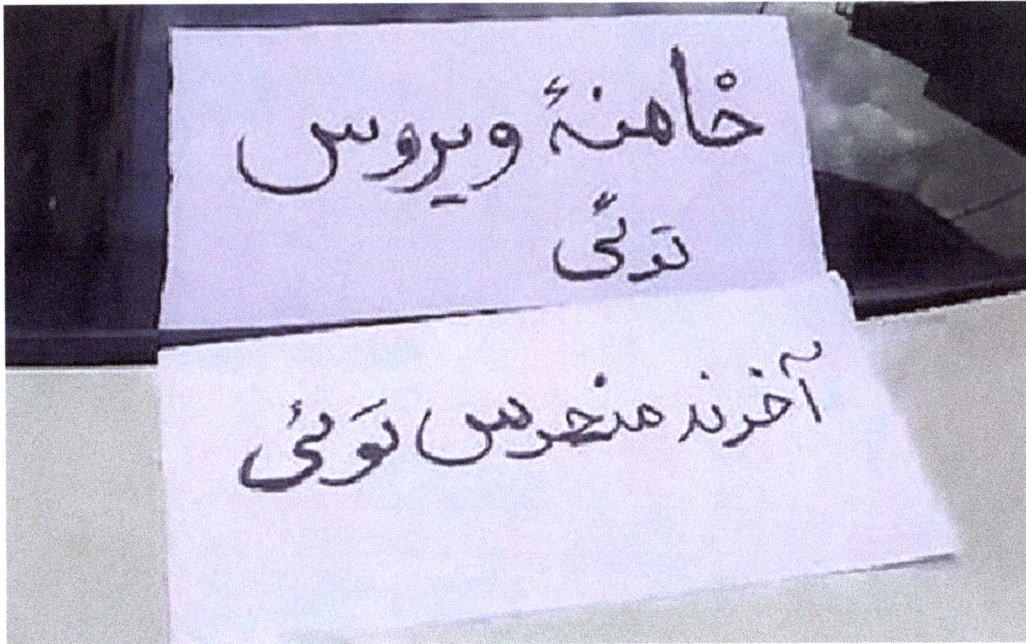

IRAN: The writing on the poster placed on a car's windshield by outraged people reads: Khamenei! you are the virus; you are the wicked mullah.

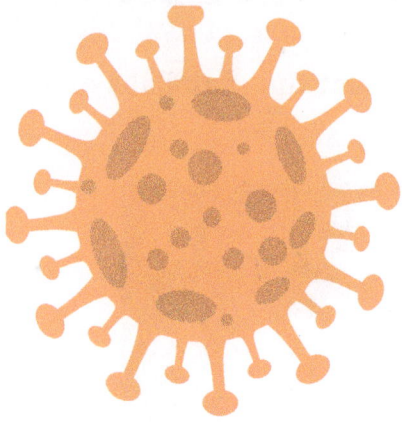

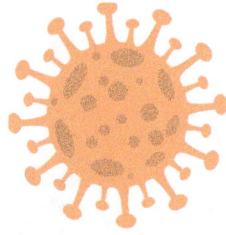

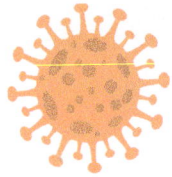

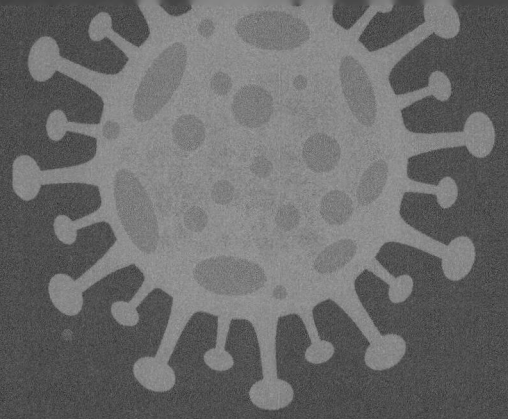

APPENDIX I

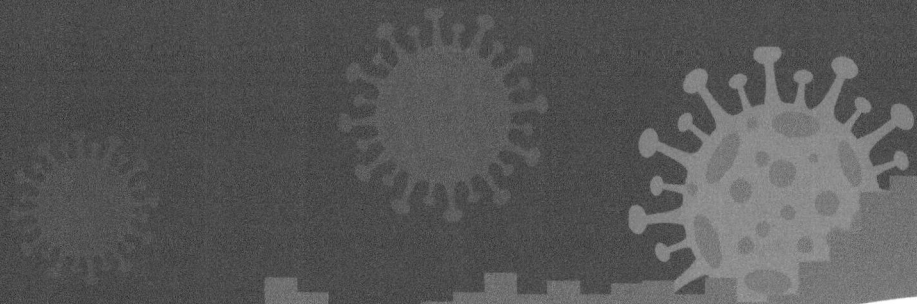

These three new documents are Mission Reports issued by the National Emergency Organization — Province of Tehran, Emergency services.

They are called "Forms for Emergency Protection Report 115." They carry the emblem of the Ministry of Health, Medical Care and Training — Center for the Management of Medical Incidents and Emergencies of the Country.

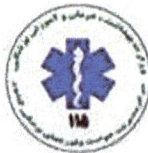

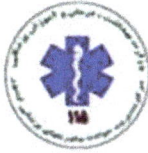

سازمان اورژانس کشور

استان تهران – اورژانس تهران

فرم گزارش مراقبت اورژانس ۱۱۵

تاریخ ماموریت : ۱۳۹۸/۱۱/۸

شماره سریال پرونده : ۷۱۳۱۵۷۲/۰۲

کرونا کد آمبولانس ۲۴۲۳

نتیجه ماموریت	مشاوره پزشکی	دارو و سرم مصرفی				اقدامات درمانی		
	پزشک تجویز کننده	نحوه تجویز	دوز	نام دارو	زمان		بعد	قبل
☑ انتقال با الزام به مرکز درمانی		-	-	-	-	☐ مانیتورینگ	☐☐	☐
☐ اقدامات اولیه و توصیه مراجعه به مرکز درمانی	-					☑ شرح حال و معاینه	☐☐	☐ CPR
☐ ماموریت کذب / ماموریت آشنا						☑ رگ گیری	☐☐	☐ پایش و کنترل خونریزی
☐ عدم حضور بیمار	دستورات :					☑ اکسیژن درمانی	☐☐	☐ لوله گذاری
☐ عدم همکاری و لغو امضا						☐ CPR	☐☐	☐ ماساژ قفسه سینه
☐ لغو از طرف مرکز هدایت و کنترل	....					☐ تکنیک سرد کردن	☐☐	☐ حمایت تنفسی
☐ تحویل به آمبولانس دیگر						☐ فیکس اندامها	☑☐	☐ VS
☐ فوت قبل از رسیدن تکنسین						☑ تکر سنتر قرآن	☐☐	☐ مشاوره لازم
☐ انتقال در حین احیا								
☐ استقرار								
☐ عدم همکاری از هر نوع اقدام درمانی								
☐ انتقال با خودروی شخصی								

برائت نامه

ایجاب خانم / آقای | شماره برائت نامه : .

علت عدم پذیرش | نام و نام خانوادگی تکنسین ارشد | نام و نام خانوادگی شاهد

محل امضا و اثر انگشت | محل امضا و اثر انگشت ارشد | محل امضا و اثر انگشت شاهد

اقلام مصرفی	توضیحات و ملاحظات ماموریت	مرکز درمانی
آنژوکت صورتی دستکش معاینه ماسک اکسیژن – بزرگسال ماسک اکسیژن یک بار مصرف کاتتر ساکشن نلکاتون رتو گاز استریل نجات	مددجو آقا ۳۷ ساله با علائم و سوابق ثبت شده که دچار سرفه و علائم سرماخوردگی دارند . اظهار میدارند که در مجاورت چین انتقال دارند و همکارانشان علائم کرونا را داشته اند و بستری میباشد علائم حیاتی چک شد معاینات نورولوژی نرمال زمان اقدامات اولیه انجام و انتقال به مرکز درمانی گردید	نام مرکز درمانی : مسیح دانشور
		تاریخ و ساعت تحویل به مرکز درمانی
		نام پزشک تحویل گیرنده
		نام پزشک تحویل گیرنده
		☐ تحویل بدون رضایت

Document Number 1: National Emergency Organization. Date of Mission: 8th of Bahman 1398 (January 28, 2020) File serial number: 7131572 Ambulance Code number: 2423.

Patient's First and Last names: Fatima Babazadeh Khameneh Nationality: Iranian Gender: Female Age: 37 Date: January 28, 2020. Address: Aghdasiyeh, Movahed Danesh Street, North Golestan Street, Laleh Alley, House number 15, Unit 401

"First responder: The lady is 37 years old, with signs of coughing, cold. She says she works at the Chinese Embassy (in Tehran), and her colleagues have had symptoms of Coronavirus. She is hospitalized. Vital signs checked. Neurology testing is normal. Initial action was taken, and she was transferred to the medical center."

Arriving at the care center: 18:34:56 pm Handing over to the care center: 19:18:01 pm Code for senior technician: 120212 Code for technician no. 1: 150081

Location: Administrative (Office) Vital Signs — checked Consultation — Given Diagnosis — done Blood Sample — Done Oxygen — Given

Name of Medical Center: Masih Daneshvar

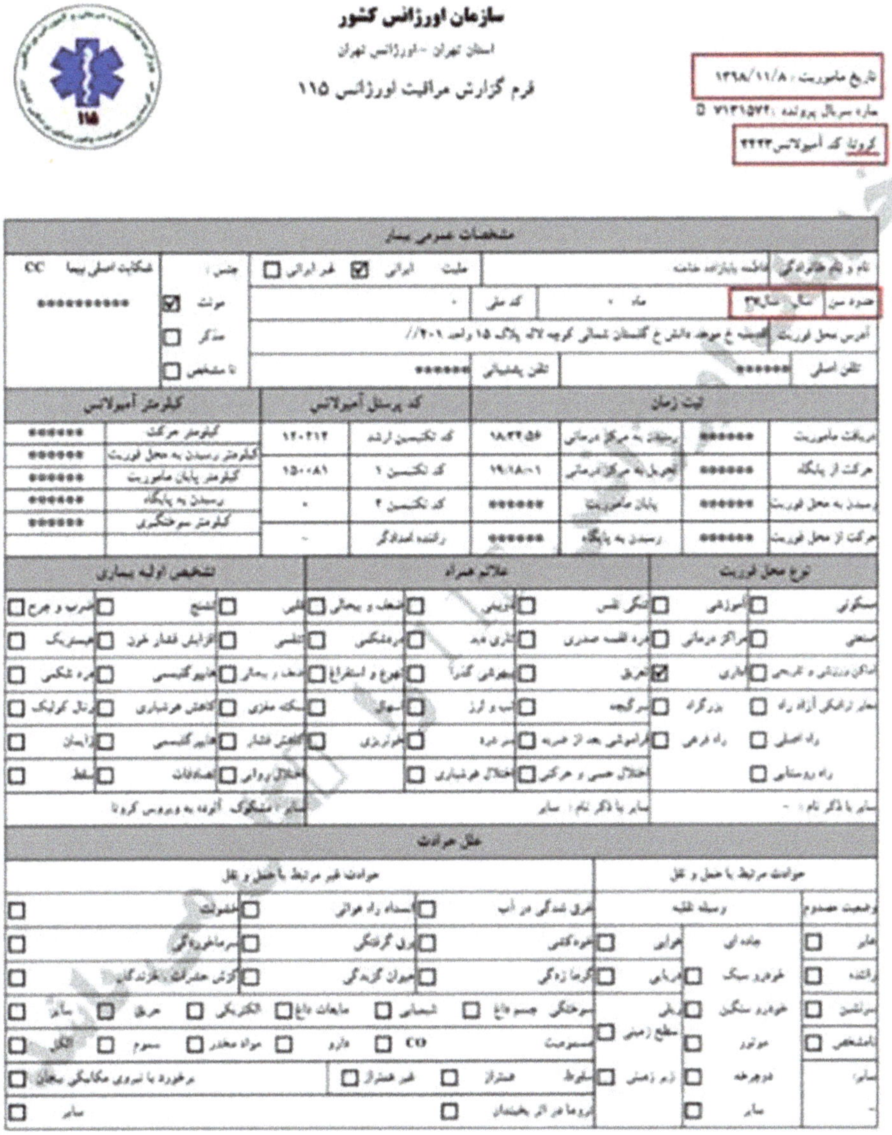

سازمان اورژانس کشور

استان تهران - اورژانس تهران

فرم گزارش مراقبت اورژانس ۱۱۵

تاریخ ماموریت : ۱۳۹۸/۱۱/۸

شماره سریال پرونده : ۷۱۳۱۵۷۲/۰۳

کرونا کد آمبولانس ۲۴۲۳

Document Number 2: National Emergency Organization. Date of Mission: 8th of Bahman 1398 (January 28, 2020) File serial number: 7131572/03

Ambulance Code number: 2423 Patient's First and Last names: Ehsan Sheikhi Nationality: Iranian Gender: Male Age: 33 Date: January 28, 2020. Address: Aghdasiyeh, Movahed Danesh Street, North Golestan Street, Laleh Alley, House number 15, Unit 401

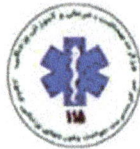

سازمان اورژانس کشور

استان تهران – اورژانس تهران

فرم گزارش مراقبت اورژانس ۱۱۵

تاریخ ماموریت : ۱۳۹۸/۱۱/۸

شماره سریال پرونده : ۷۱۲۱۵۷۲

کد آمبولانس ۲۴۲۳

نتیجه ماموریت	مشاوره پزشکی	دارو و سرم مصرفی					اقدامات درمانی				
	کد پزشک	نحوه تجویز	دوز	نام دارو	زمان	بعد	قبل	حین			قبل
☑ انتقال یا اعزام به مرکز درمانی	-	-	-	-	-	مانیتورینگ ☐	☐☐		ساکشن ☐
☐ اقدامات اولیه و توصیه مراجعه به مرکز درمانی	-	-	-	-	-	☑ شرح حال و معاینه	☐☐		CPR
☐ ماموریت کنسل / ماموریت کاذب	-	-	-	-	-	☑ رگ گیری	☐☐		باندپی و کنترل خونریزی ☐
☐ عدم حضور بیمار	دستورات :	-	-	-	-	☑ اکسیژن درمانی	☐☐		لوله گذاری ☐
☐ عدم همکاری و اخذ امضا	●●●●●●●●●	-	-	-	-	☐ CBR	☐☐		ماساژ قفسه سینه ☐
☐ لغو از طرف مرکز هدایت و کنترل		-	-	-	-	☑	☐☐		حمایت تنفسی ☐
☐ تحویل به آمبولانس دیگر		-	-	-	-	☑ فیکس اندامها	☑☐		VS ☐
☐ فوت قبل از رسیدن تکنسین		-	-	-	-	☑ تکنر سنتر اطراف	☑☐		مشاوره لازم ☐
☐ فوت در حین احیا		-	-	-	-				
☐ استقرار									
☐ عدم همکاری از هر نوع اقدام درمانی		-	-	-	-				
☐ انتقال با خودروی شخصی		-	-	-	-				

برائت نامه

اینجانب خانم/آقای

شماره برائت نامه : -

نام و نام خانوادگی شاهد	نام و نام خانوادگی تکنسین ارشد	علت عدم پذیرش
محل امضا و اثر انگشت شاهد	محل امضا و اثر انگشت ارشد	محل امضا و اثر انگشت

اقلام مصرفی	توضیحات و ملاحظات ماموریت	مرکز درمانی
آنژیوکت صورتی-دستکش معاینه-ماسک-چسب ملحفه-برانکاردینه نجات-کانولای بینی	مذمجم خانم ۳۳ساله با علائم و سوابق ثبت شده که دچار سرفه و علائم سرماخوردگی دارند. اظهار مبدارند در سفارت چین اشتغال دارند و همکارانشان علائم کرونا را داشته اند و بستری میباشد علائم حیاتی چک شد معاینات نورولوژی نرمال اقدامات اولیه انجام و انتقال به مرکز درمانی گردید	نام مرکز درمانی مسیح دانشور
		تاریخ و ساعت تحویل به مرکز درمانی
		نام پزشک تحویل گیرنده
		کد پزشک تحویل گیرنده
		☐ تحویل بدون رضایت

"First responder: He is 33 years old, with coughing, and symptoms of cold. He says he works at the Chinese Embassy (in Tehran), and his colleagues have had symptoms of Coronavirus. He is hospitalized. Vital signs checked. Neurology testing is normal. Initial action was taken, and he was transferred to the medical center."

Arriving at the care center: 18:34:56 pm Handing over to the care center: 19:18:01 pm Code for senior technician: 120212 Code for technician no. 1: 150081

Location: Administrative (Office) VS — checked Consultation — Given Diagnosis — done Blood Sample — Done Oxygen — Given

Name of Medical Center: Masih Daneshvar

سازمان اورژانس کشور

استان تهران - اورژانس تهران

فرم گزارش مراقبت اورژانس ۱۱۵

تاریخ ماموریت : ۱۳۹۸/۱۱/۸

شماره سریال پرونده :۷۱۳۱۵۷۲/۰۲

کرونا کد آمبولانس ۲۴۲۳

مشخصات عمومی بیمار				
نام و نام خانوادگی	محمدعلی ذوالقدرنیا	ملیت ایرانی ☑ غیر ایرانی ☐	جنس :	شکایت اصلی بیمار CC
حدود سن سال: سال۳۳	ماه ۰	کد ملی ۰	مونث ☐	**********
آدرس محل فوریت	اقدسیه خ موحد دانش خ گلستان شمالی کوچه لاله پلاک ۱۵ واحد ۴۰۱//		مذکر ☑	
تلفن اصلی	******	تلفن پشتیبانی ******	نامشخص ☐	

ثبت زمان				کد پرسنل آمبولانس		کیلومتر آمبولانس	
دریافت ماموریت	******	رسیدن به مرکز درمانی	۱۸:۳۴:۵۶	کد تکنسین ارشد	۱۲۰۲۱۲	کیلومتر حرکت	******
حرکت از پایگاه	******	تحویل به مرکز درمانی	۱۹:۱۸:۰۱	کد تکنسین ۱	۱۵۰۰۸۱	کیلومتر رسیدن به محل فوریت	******
رسیدن به محل فوریت	******	پایان ماموریت	******	کد تکنسین ۲	۰	کیلومتر پایان ماموریت	******
حرکت از محل فوریت	******	رسیدن به پایگاه	******	راننده امدادگر	-	رسیدن به پایگاه	******
						کیلومتر سوختگیری	******

نوع محل فوریت		علائم همراه			تشخیص اولیه بیماری		
مسکونی ☐	آموزشی ☐	تنگی نفس ☐	بیهوشی ☐	ضعف و بیحالی ☐	قلبی ☐	تشنج ☐	ضرب و جرح ☐
صنعتی ☐	مراکز درمانی ☐	درد قفسه صدری ☐	تاری دید ☐	رنگپریدگی ☐	تنفسی ☐	افزایش فشار خون ☐	هیستریک ☐
اماکن ورزشی و تفریحی ☐	اداری ☐	تعریق ☑	بیهوشی گذرا ☐	تهوع و استفراغ ☐	ضعف و بیحالی ☐	هایپوگلیسمی ☐	درد شکمی ☐
معابر ترافیکی آزاد راه ☐	بزرگراه ☐	سرگیجه ☐	تب و لرز ☐	سرفه ☐	سکته مغزی ☐	کاهش هوشیاری ☐	رنال کولیک ☐
راه اصلی ☐	راه فرعی ☐	فراموشی بعد از ضربه ☐	سردرد ☐	خونریزی ☐	کاهش فشار ☐	هایپرگلیسمی ☐	زایمان ☐
راه روستایی ☐		اختلال حسی و حرکتی ☐	اختلال هوشیاری ☐		اختلال روانی ☐	تصادفات ☐	سقط ☐
سایر با ذکر نام : -		سایر با ذکر نام : سایر			سایر : مشکوک آلوده به ویروس کرونا		

علل حوادث				
حوادث مرتبط با حمل و نقل			حوادث غیر مرتبط با حمل و نقل	
وضعیت مصدوم	وسیله نقلیه			
عابر ☐	جاده ای	هوایی ☐	خودکشی ☐	برق گرفتگی ☐ / سرمازدگی ☐
راننده ☐	خودرو سبک ☐	دریایی ☐	گرمازدگی ☐	حیوان گزیدگی ☐ / گزش حشرات، خزندگان ☐
سرنشین ☐	خودرو سنگین ☐	ریلی ☐	سوختگی: جسم داغ ☐ شیمیایی ☐ مایعات داغ ☐ الکتریکی ☐ حریق ☐ سایر ☐	
نامشخص ☐	موتور ☐	سطح زمینی ☐	مسمومیت: CO ☐ دارو ☐ مواد مخدر ☐ سموم ☐ الکل ☐	
سایر: -	دوچرخه ☐	زیر زمینی ☐	سقوط: عمدی ☐ غیر عمدی ☐	برخورد با نیروی مکانیکی بیجان ☐
	سایر ☐		تروما در اثر بیهوشی ☐	سایر ☐
			غرق شدگی در آب ☐	انسداد راه هوایی ☐ / خشونت ☐

Document Number 3: National Emergency Organization. Date of Mission: 8th of Bahman 1398 (January 28, 2020) File serial number: 7131572/02 Ambulance Code number: 2423 Patient's First and Last names: Mohammad Ali Zolqadrnia Nationality: Iranian Gender: Male Age: 33 Date: January 28, 2020. Address: Aghdasiyeh, Movahed Danesh Street, North Golestan Street, Laleh Alley, House number 15, Unit 401

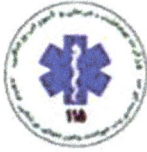

سازمان اورژانس کشور

استان تهران - اورژانس تهران

فرم گزارش مأموریت اورژانس ۱۱۵

تاریخ مأموریت : ۱۳۹۸/۱۱/۸

شماره سریال پرونده : ۷۱۲۱۵۷۲/۰۲

کرونا کد آمبولانس ۲۴۲۳

"First responder: He is 33 years old, with sever coughing, symptoms of cold. He says he was in China for the past 12 days, and in the first three days after arriving in Tehran, he had high fever, diarrhea, and sever coughing. He says he works at the Chinese Embassy (in Tehran), and his colleagues have had symptoms of Coronavirus. He is hospitalized. Vital signs checked. Neurology testing is normal. Initial action was taken, and he was transferred to the medical center."

Arriving at the care center: 18:34:56 pm Handing over to the care center: 19:18:01 pm Code for senior technician: 120212 Code for technician no. 1: 150081

Location: Administrative (Office) VS — checked Consultation — Given Diagnosis — done Blood Sample — Done Oxygen — Given

Name of Medical Center: Masih Daneshvar

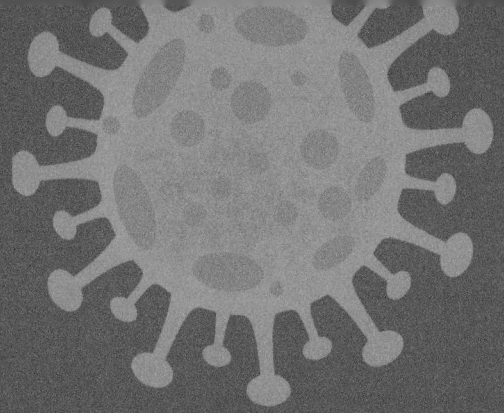

Appendix II

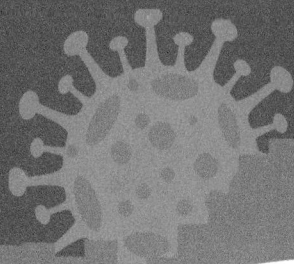

A brief description of several the regime's economic powerhouses

"SETAD"

"SETAD" refers to the Headquarters for Executing the Order of the Imam.[37] A Reuters investigation published on November 11, 2013, which was the result of a six-month investigation, estimated its assets at about $95 billion. According to Reuters, the $95B figure comes from analyzing official statements by SETAD authorities, figures obtained from the Tehran stock exchange, company websites, and information from the US Treasury.

Setad is comprised of two main components, the first of which includes its primary investments and properties, buildings and real-estate confiscated from religious minorities, dissidents and opponents — properties that the regime views as being "without owners."

In 1991, Khamenei issued an order that empowered Setad to confiscate not only properties that belonged to monarchists but also the assets of Jews, Bahais, and other religious minorities that had migrated to other countries, as well as Muslim emigrants whose assets were left without a power of attorney or supervisors. In the years since, the mission and scope of activities of SETAD have expanded significantly. Later, confiscated assets whose ownership was contested, without inheritors, or abandoned were added to SETAD's portfolio. Reuters estimated that this portion of SETAD's portfolio is worth about $52B.[38]

The second portion of SETAD's holdings includes shares in large companies. This financial mafia network is now controlling the big companies using Supreme Leader Ali Khamenei's authority. The value of these assets is upwards of $43B.

---

37 *Iran: The Rise of the Revolutionary Guards Financial Empire: How the Supreme Leader and IRGC Rob the People to Fund International Terror* (Washington, D. C.: National Council of Resistance of Iran, 2017) , p.76

38 Steve Stecklow, Babak Dehghanpisheh, and Yeganeh Torbati, "Reuters Investigates — Assets of the Ayatollah," Reuters (Thomson Reuters, November 11, 2013), https://www.reuters.com/investigates/iran/#article/part1

In 2007, the mullahs' parliament (*Majlis*) passed a law according to which centers and organizations affiliated with the "Leadership" (Khamenei) cannot be subjected to any investigation or research unless it is authorized by Khamenei himself.

On June 17, 2013, the head of the mullahs' Judiciary, Sadeq Larijani, issued a directive to the regime's judges and courts, which said in part: "With respect to assets left over by those accused in cases concerning Article 49 of the Constitution, where rulings have been made in favor of other institutions but so far have not taken steps to identify, supervise or take ownership, the courts are obligated to review these matters and take steps to issue final rulings in favor of the Setad-e Ejraee Imam [SETAD]."[39]

Therefore, two branches of the regime, the Judiciary and Legislative, have condoned the absolute and unconditional theft and confiscation of people's properties by the institution of the Supreme Leader.

Khamenei has appointed mullah Hossein-Ali Nayyeri, the head of the death commission in Tehran during the 1988 massacre of thousands of political prisoners, as chairman of the board of directors of SETAD and, therefore, its highest official.

In June 2013, the US Treasury announced the identification and sanctioning of SETAD and a network of 37 related companies that secretly make investments on behalf of the Iranian regime.[40]

Setad has set up several so-called "foundations" to cover up its activities. One of them is called the Barekat Foundation, which is active in various financial and commercial enterprises. It has a drug company called Barekat Pharmaceuticals, which controls over 20 subsidiaries. In 2011, it had revenues upwards of one billion dollars. Based on this one entity, one can only guess the scope of Khamenei's vast economic cartel.

Moreover, the Etemad Mobin Development company, 38% of whose shares are controlled by Setad, purchased more than half of Iran's telecommunications

---

39 Iran Students' News Agency (ISNA News Agency, June 17, 2013), accessed April 4, 2020, https://bit.ly/39LmgWn

40 "U.S. Department of the Treasury," Treasury Targets Assets of Iranian Leadership, March 27, 2020, https://www.treasury.gov/press-center/press-releases/Pages/jl1968.aspx

company for 7,800 billion Tomans (at the time about $8B) a few years ago. Subsequent to the purchase, one of SETAD's senior-ranking officials was appointed as the head of the telecommunications company of Iran. Companies and foundations related to this cartel are constantly signing contracts and deals worth hundreds of millions and at times billions of dollars within the regime.

Astan-e Qods Razavi

Astan-e Qods Razavi is the largest endowment institution in the Islamic world.[41] The organization and management of all the religious ceremonies and financial gifts for the shrine of the eighth Shiite Imam over the past several centuries have been controlled by the Astan-e Qods, whose head is directly appointed by the Supreme Leader. Over the past 42 years, three people have been handpicked by Khamenei to run this vast institution: Mullah Abbas Vaez Tabasi who died in March 2016; Ebrahim Raisi, current head of Khamenei's Judiciary and member of the death commission during the 1988 massacre in Iran; and mullah Ahmad Marvi, a close Khamenei confidant. No one other than Khamenei himself has the authority to hold this economic powerhouse accountable.

Astan-e Qods employs tens of thousands of workers. It is also completely tax-exempt. It has more than 50 large companies. 43% of the land base (over 13,000 hectares) of Mashad (the second most populous city in Iran) is owned by Astan. In addition to Mashhad, Astan has land, gardens, wells, water channels and over 300,000 renters across Iran, including in the provinces of Hamedan, Eastern Azerbaijan, Golestan, Gilan, Tehran, Semnan and Yazd. Large swathes of land, with an estimated value of over $20B, are owned by this foundation.

This is in addition to the array of its other assets. Astan has complete and independent control in oil fields related to its operations. It has exclusive oil rigs and has full independent authority for importing or exporting oil from areas under its control. Ownership of a portion of the railway, heavy and foundational industries such as the Mobarakeh Steel company, and large portions of mines and natural resources are owned by Astan-e Qods. For the past few years, Astan has also become involved in projects outside Iran, including operations by its subsidiaries.

---

41   *Iran: The Rise of the Revolutionary Guards Financial Empire: How the Supreme Leader and IRGC Rob the People to Fund International Terror* (Washington, D. C.: National Council of Resistance of Iran, 2017) , p.84

These include building railway bridges on the Euphrates river, with an estimated length of 1,000 meters, in Syria.

Astan also controls 10% of the total production of sugar cubes, 11% of decorative stones, 3.7% of urban and transport buses, and one-sixth of bread in the entire country.

Every year, the companies affiliated with Astan produce 73,000 tons of dried milk, 300 tons of red meat, 1,000 tons of white meat, 100,000 tons of agricultural products, 10 million square meters of fabric, and 6,000 square meters of hand-woven carpet. On an annual basis, it also completes more than 136 construction projects, development projects, road building and urban initiatives.

49% of the shares of the Razavi oil and gas development company are owned by Astan-e Qods. The remaining 51% are owned by the Social Security Investment Company. This company develops oil and gas fields and is active in the commerce of oil and oil-based products. It also invests in oil and gas and petrochemical products. Among its projects was the building of five offshore drilling rigs in 2015. According to its CEO, it has signed a $1.1B oil and gas contract.

The Mostazafan Foundation

The Mostazafan Foundation is controlled by the Supreme Leader and governed through a board of directors. The foundation oversees close to 140 companies in the food, chemical, petrochemical, metals, building, agricultural and tourism industries. Owing to its special legal status, it can work directly with foreign companies.[42]

In the past, the Mostazafan Foundation was considered the largest economic powerhouse in Iran. Today, it has over 200,000 employees.[43]

In 1997, the former head of Mostazafan, Mohsen Rafiqdoost, said: "The Mostazafan Foundation has about 400 commercial companies, and produces 28% of the

---

42 In the past, in 1989, Mostazafan Foundation controlled over 800 companies and commercial entities, all of which were confiscated properties. After the so-called privatization and transfer of state assets to private entities, the number of these companies was reduced to 400 in 1999.

43 *Iran: The Rise of the Revolutionary Guards Financial Empire: How the Supreme Leader and IRGC Rob the People to Fund International Terror* (Washington, D. C.: National Council of Resistance of Iran, 2017) , p.81

country's textiles, 22% of cement, about 45% of non-alcoholic beverages, 28% of tires, and 25% of Iran's sugar."[44] In 2009, the foundation owned almost 140 companies in total, including the Sina Bank. The Zamzam company, Alavi Foundation and the Behran oil company are also among the foundation's assets.[45] Based on its official financial statements in 2016, the foundation's assets are worth about $14B. In fact, the company's real net worth is considered to be several-fold higher.

The financial statements of 2016 claimed revenues of about $7B. Approximately 35% of this amount resulted from the sale of products, primarily in the food and agricultural sectors, oil and gas, and industries and mining. Approximately 65% of the revenues result from provision of services in the financial and banking sectors and communication technologies, and industries and mining. Declared net profits in 2016 were $700M. The annual retained earnings have been estimated at about $5.3B.

Khatam al-Anbiya Construction Headquarters

The Khatam al-Anbiya Construction Headquarters is the main financial and commercial arm of the Islamic Revolutionary Guard Corps (IRGC). It began its activities as a contractor of industrial and construction projects following the ceasefire in the Iran-Iraq War in 1989. Khatam is the largest contractor for government projects in Iran. It has 5,000 subcontractors and about 135,000 employees.[46] For years, Khatam has not limited its activities to specific fields and does not accept projects less than about $25M. Its projects have included the Sadr highway project in Tehran, the South Pars phases 15 and 16, the Gatvand dam construction, various highways, and different vast tunnels. In the oil sector, on March 15, 2010, the Oil Ministry signed a $850M contract for pipelines with Khatam's Qorb. Later, the National Iranian Gas Company awarded a project for the construction of a 270 km pipeline worth about $250M to the Khatam company. The first phase of this project was also previously awarded to Khatam in 2006 and was worth $1.3B.[47]

---

44 Jaras, July 5, 2010, accessed April 5, 2020, https://bit.ly/3bYiiet

45 *Iran: The Rise of the Revolutionary Guards Financial Empire: How the Supreme Leader and IRGC Rob the People to Fund International Terror* (Washington, D. C.: National Council of Resistance of Iran, 2017)

46 IRGC Brig. Gen. Abadollah Abdollahi, then-commander of Khatam al-Anbiya, state-run Sharq Daily, December 17, 2014

47 "Awarding new oil projects worth $850M to Khatam al-Anbiya," State-Run Abrar daily, March 16, 2007

A plan by the government of former president Mahmoud Ahmadinejad anticipated taking water from the Caspian Sea and transferring it to Semnan Province. This project was awarded to Khatam, and more than $150M in credit was reserved for it. The plan was supposed to transfer 500 million cubic meters of water from the Caspian Sea through pipelines and canals to Semnan Province and the Lut desert. The funding was transferred to the IRGC's accounts, but nothing actually happened on the ground.

The development projects for natural gas phases for South Pars 15 and 16 in August 2006 were awarded to Khatam without a formal procurement process. The contract was worth over $2B. The Ahmadinejad government's conduct in awarding large projects to military institutions and Khatam turned the Khatam company into one of the biggest contractors and builders in Iran.[48] Rostam Qassemi, former commander of Khatam (and former Ahmadinejad Oil Minister and head of Qods Force logistics in Syria), has said that the investment for South Pars phases 15 and 16 joint gas fields depended on securing one billion dollars from foreign reserves.

Social Security Investment Company

On December 18, 2019, the state-run daily *Farheekhtegan* published a shocking economic report: "Information accessible from 15 banks showed that the fixtures and bank obligations of 456 legal persons and entities amounted to $89.6B, equivalent to the government's budget in 2020. State companies like the National Oil Company and the Social Security Investment Company had the largest share of bank loans. They received these loans not to expand domestic production but to pay for their day-to-day operations. The majority of the loans related to 20 to 30 companies and legal entities."[49]

The Social Security Investment Company is a holding company belonging to the Social Security Organization. The company is active in investments, commerce, trade, management and investment banking.

The Social Security Investment Company was established by the Social Security Organization as a special investment arm with an initial capital of close to

48   State-run Abrar daily, April 19, 2010

49   Farhikhtegan daily, December 18, 2019, accessed April 4, 2020, https://bit.ly/2Xfhs8R

$500,000. Six years ago, close to 10% of all the value of the Tehran Stock Exchange belonged to the company's subsidiaries.[50]

It is worth mentioning that the revenues and profits of this company have been on the rise.

The Social Security Investment Company has multiple subsidiaries, including the Daroupakhsh Pharma factories, Exir Pharma, Farabi Pharma, Faka agriculture and free-range company, Zahravi Pharma, Abu Reyhan Pharma, Caspian Pharma, Dana Pharma, Razek Laboratories, Pars Pharma, and Gelatin Capsule Iran Company.

According to the state-run ILNA, the company's profits are astronomical: "The profits of the Social Security Investment Company at the end of the financial calendar year (March 2019) were more than $2B, which compared to the previous year showed a 213% increase. The company's net profits at the end of the financial calendar year (March 2019) reached $6.7B, which marks a 286% increase compared to the same period the year before. It is interesting to note that the rate of return of the company in the current year has been 18%, which is an 8-fold growth compared to the same period last year. Moreover, the economic conduct of the company over the past nine months and the jump in its activities paint a very bright picture for its companies in 2020, resulting in a growth in production. On this basis, there have been sales of over $1.3B, which shows a 60% increase compared to the previous year. Net profits have been $6B, showing an increase of 141% compared to the previous year."

The National Development Fund

Another monetary source for the clerical regime worth tens of billions of dollars is the National Development Fund. This fund was set up to invest in the regime's long-term economic projects, but the authority over its spending rests with Supreme Leader Ali Khamenei. The latest report on the fund came out on March 26, 2020, when urgent medical needs were expressed. The regime's TV channel said: "The total medical requirements and the amount that this unemployment insurance fund needs are one billion dollars. God willing, we

50 Alef News Site, August 2, 2014, accessed April 4, 2020, https://bit.ly/3bXIoym

will write this letter today and we hope His Excellency the Supreme Leader agrees to draw a billion dollars from this fund to allocate to the challenges of the coronavirus, especially in the area of medicine and treatment, which are desperately needed, both in terms of equipping hospitals and other related initiatives."[51]

Since the coronavirus epidemic in Iran, some of the regime's officials have pointed to the reserves in the National Development Fund to address medical needs, but these concerns have not been addressed to date.[52]

According to the state-run daily *Etemad*, "Since the second decade of the current century, the National Development Fund has been set up to save a portion of the annual revenues from oil and byproducts exports in order to support future generations and the country's development. During these years, based on what was determined in the five-year plan, the government was obligated to pay into the fund. According to the fifth development plan, 20% was to be added to the fund in the first year and after that an annual rate of three percent was to be added. For the sixth plan of development, 30% of oil revenues must be allocated to the fund and an additional two percent must be deposited annually."[53]

As for the money available in this secretive fund, during his early years, Rouhani announced at Tehran University that the coffers were completely empty (October 14, 2013) . However, his remarks were met with widespread criticism and later Ahmad Tavakkoli announced that there was $15B in the fund. The head of the fund said that it had $42B and the chair of the inspections organization of the country at the time, Nasser Seraj, said $54.5B was available. The head of the Central Bank during Ahmadinejad's presidency, Mahmoud Bahmani, said after Rouhani's speech: "The country's foreign reserve exceeds $100B, and there is $32B to $34B available in the National Development Fund. …. Some reports estimate that the reserve is closer to $90B."[54]

---

51   Fararu, March 26, 2020, https://bit.ly/39LJMlQ

52   Etemad Online, March 7, 2020, accessed April 5, 2020, https://bit.ly/34acj3o

53   Ibid.

54   peykeiran.com, February 4, 2020, accessed April 4, 2020, https://bit.ly/2XcocEt

Following the elimination of the regime's chief terrorist and Commander of the extraterritorial Qods Force, Qassem Soleimani, the regime's Parliamentary Speaker, Ali Larijani, said that the government had awarded $200M to the Qods Force from the National Development Fund on the orders of Khamenei.

Prior to that, the government's public relations office had said that $2B euros from the same fund would be allocated to "defense-related" matters. In previous years, the regime has followed a similar pattern, dedicating a portion of the fund to the defense budget.[55]

---

55   peykeiran.com, February 4, 2020, accessed April 4, 2020, https://bit.ly/2XcocEt

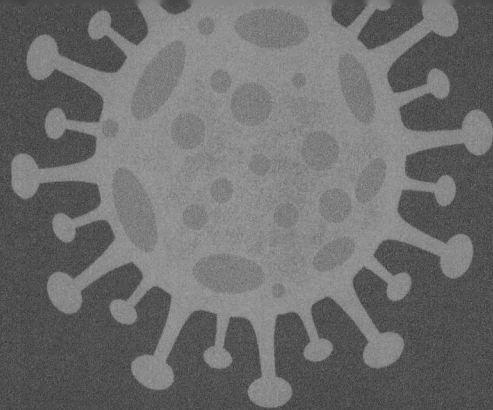

Appendix III

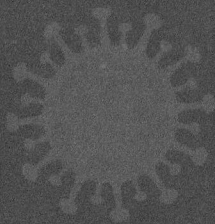
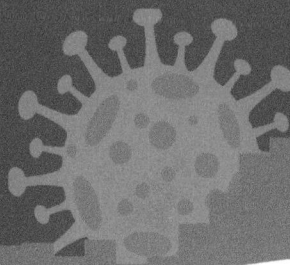

CORONAVIRUS DEATH TOLL
(AS OF MAY 8, 2020):

According to the figures tallied by the Mujahedin-e Khalq (PMOI/MEK) main opposition movement, based on information from its sources in hospitals across the country, the real death toll in 314 towns and cities in all 31 provinces of Iran has exceeded 40,000.

PROVINCE	DEATH TOLL	AS OF
Tehran	6,690	08-May-20
Qom	3,290	07-May-20
Khorassan Razavi	2,935	08-May-20
Gilan	2,690	07-May-20
Isfahan	2,470	08-May-20
Mazandaran	2,480	08-May-20
Khuzestan	2,055	08-May-20
East Azerbaijan	1,450	26-Apr-20
Alborz	1,599	08-May-20
West Azerbaijan	1,215	07-May-20
Golestan	1,235	03-May-20
Kermanshah	960	04-May-20
Hamedan	985	07-May-20
Fars	1,005	06-May-20
Lorestan	1,030	08-May-20
Sistan and Baluchestan	1,091	07-May-20
Ardabil	670	26-Apr-20
Semnan	910	05-May-20
Kurdistan	640	06-May-20
Yazd	690	05-May-20
Markazi	535	08-May-20
Zanjan	485	30-Apr-20
Qazvin	445	06-May-20
Kerman	435	05-May-20
North Khorasan	442	08-May-20
Bushehr	435	06-May-20
Chaharmahal and Bakhtiari	330	05-May-20
Ilam	270	01-May-20
Kohgiluyeh and Boyer-Ahmad	255	05-May-20
South Khorasan	135	07-May-20
Hormozgan	163	06-May-20

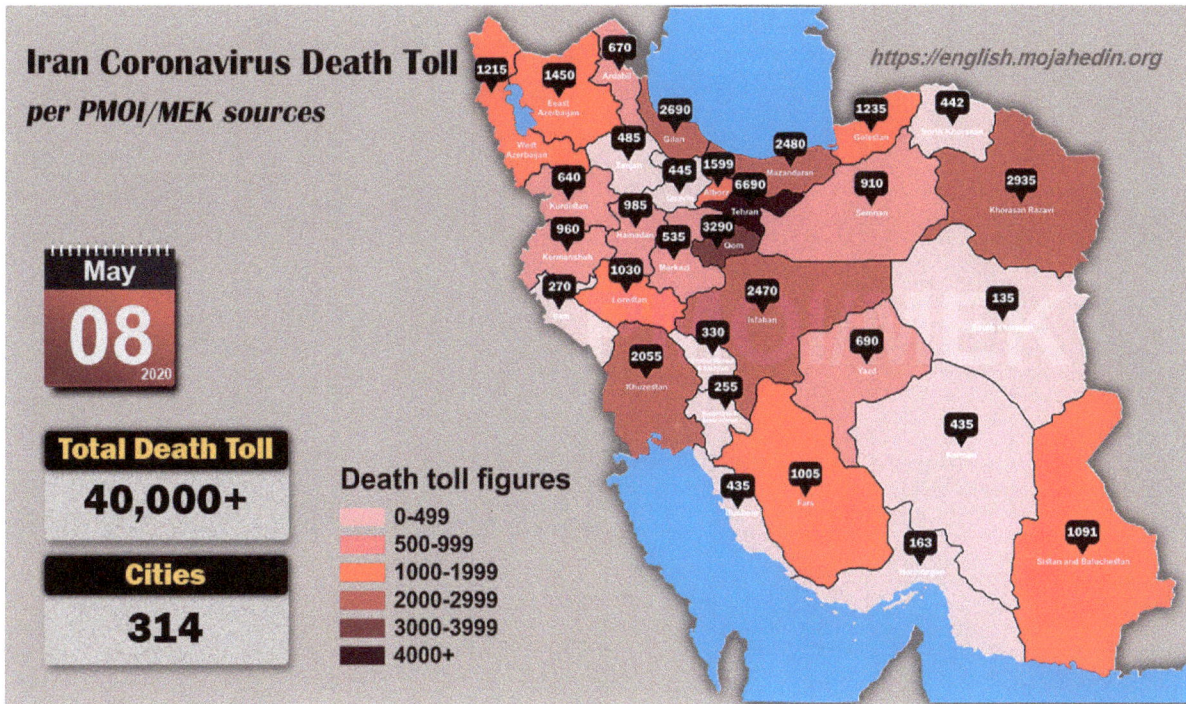

Iran Coronavirus Death Toll

per PMOI/MEK sources

https://english.mojahedin.org

May 08 2020

Total Death Toll
40,000+

Cities
314

Death toll figures
- 0-499
- 500-999
- 1000-1999
- 2000-2999
- 3000-3999
- 4000+

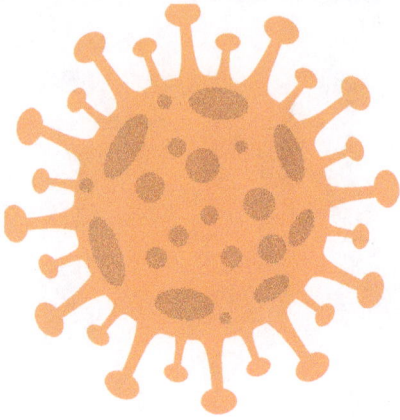

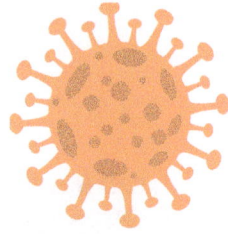

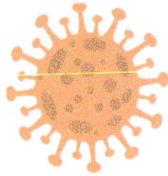

List of publications

List of Publications by the National Council of Resistance of Iran, U.S. Representative Office

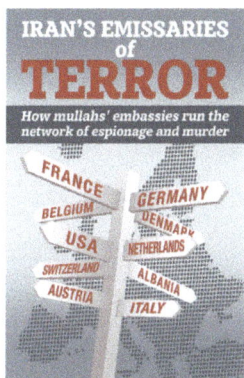

Iran's Emissaries of Terror

June 2019, 208 pages

This book explains the extent to which Tehran's embassies and diplomats are at the core of both the planning and execution of international terrorism targeting Iranian dissidents, as well as central to Tehran's direct and proxy terrorism against other countries.

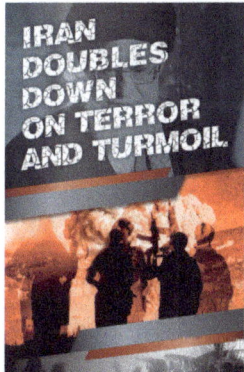

Iran Doubles Down on Terror and Turmoil

November 2018, 63 pages

This book examines the regime's political and economic strategy, which revolves around terrorism and physical annihilation of opponents. Failing to quell growing popular protests, Tehran has bolstered domestic suppression with blatant terrorism and intimidation.

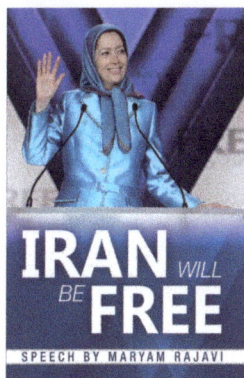

Iran Will Be Free:
Speech by Maryam Rajavi

September 2018, 54 pages

Text of a keynote speech delivered by Mrs. Maryam Rajavi on June 30, 2018, at the Iranian Resistance's grand gathering in Paris, France explaining the path to freedom in Iran and what she envisions for future Iran.

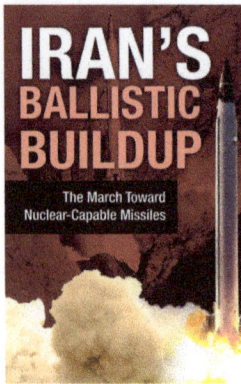

Iran's Ballistic Buildup: The March Toward Nuclear-Capable Missiles

May 2018, 136 pages

This manuscript surveys Iran's missile capabilities, including the underlying organization, structure, production, and development infrastructure, as well as launch facilities and the command centers. The book exposes the nexus between the regime's missile activities and its nuclear weapons program, including ties with North Korea.

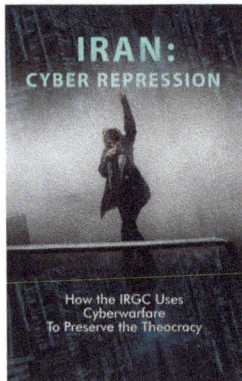

Iran: Cyber Repression: How the IRGC Uses Cyberwarfare to Preserve the Theocracy

February 2018, 70 pages

This manuscript demonstrates how the Iranian regime, under the supervision and guidance of the IRGC and the Ministry of Intelligence and Security (MOIS), have employed new cyberwarfare and tactics in a desperate attempt to counter the growing dissent inside the country.

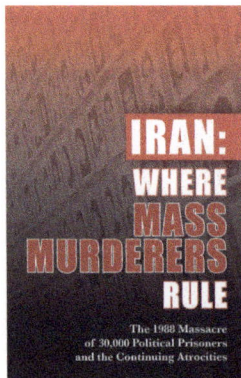

Iran: Where Mass Murderers Rule: The 1988 Massacre of 30,000 Political Prisoners and the Continuing Atrocities

November 2017, 161 pages

Iran: Where Mass Murderers Rule is an expose of the current rulers of Iran and their track record in human rights violations. The book details how 30,000 political prisoners fell victim to politicide during the summer of 1988 and showcases the egregious political extinction of a group of people.

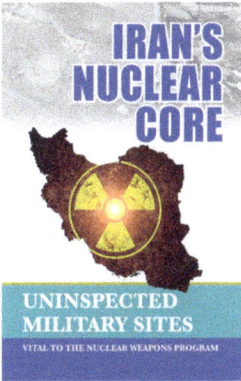

Iran's Nuclear Core: Uninspected Military Sites, Vital to the Nuclear Weapons Program

October 2017, 52 pages

This book details how the nuclear weapons program is at the heart of, and not parallel to, the civil nuclear program of Iran. The program has been run by the Islamic Revolutionary Guards Corp (IRGC) since the beginning, and the main nuclear sites and nuclear research facilities have been hidden from the eyes of the United Nations nuclear watchdog.

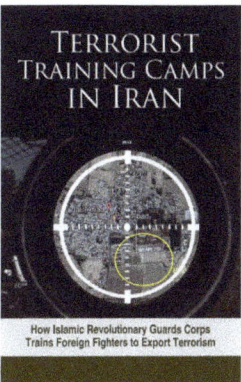

Terrorist Training Camps in Iran: How Islamic Revolutionary Guards Corps Trains Foreign Fighters to Export Terrorism

June 2017, 56 pages

The book details how Islamic Revolutionary Guards Corps trains foreign fighters in 15 various camps in Iran to export terrorism. The IRGC has created a large directorate within its extraterritorial arm, the Quds Force, in order to expand its training of foreign mercenaries as part of the strategy to step up its meddling abroad in Syria, Iraq, Yemen, Bahrain, Afghanistan and elsewhere.

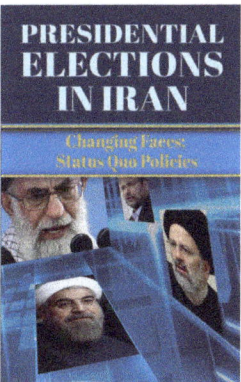

Presidential Elections in Iran: Changing Faces; Status Quo Policies

May 2017, 78 pages

The book reviews the past 11 presidential elections, demonstrating that the only criterion for qualifying as a candidate is practical and heartfelt allegiance to the Supreme Leader. An unelected vetting watchdog, the Guardian Council makes that determination.

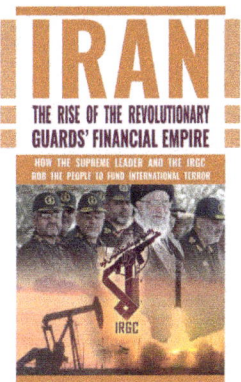

The Rise of Iran's Revolutionary Guards' Financial Empire: How the Supreme Leader and the IRGC Rob the People to Fund International Terror

March 2017, 174 pages

This study shows how ownership of property in various spheres of the economy is gradually shifted from the population writ large towards a minority ruling elite comprised of the Supreme Leader's office and the IRGC, using 14 powerhouses, and how the money ends up funding terrorism worldwide.

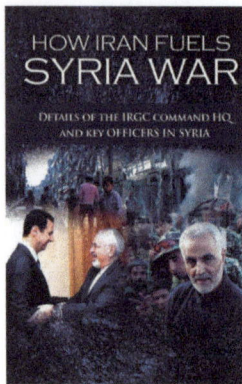

How Iran Fuels Syria War: Details of the IRGC Command HQ and Key Officers in Syria

November 2016, 74 pages

This book examines how the Iranian regime has effectively engaged in the military occupation of Syria by marshaling 70,000 forces, including the Islamic Revolutionary Guard Corps (IRGC) and mercenaries from other countries into Syria; is paying monthly salaries to over 250,000 militias and agents to prolong the conflict; and divided the country into 5 zones of conflict, establishing 18 command, logistics and operations centers.

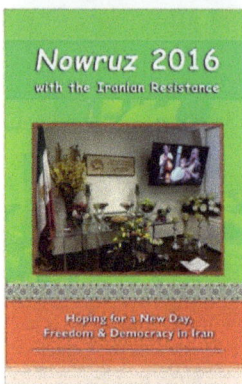

Nowruz 2016 with the Iranian Resistance: Hoping for a New Day, Freedom and Democracy in Iran

April 2016, 36 pages

This book describes Iranian New Year, Nowruz celebrations at the Washington office of Iran's parliament-in-exile, the National Council of Resistance of Iran. The yearly event marks the beginning of spring. It includes select speeches by dignitaries who have attended the NCRIUS Nowruz celebrations.

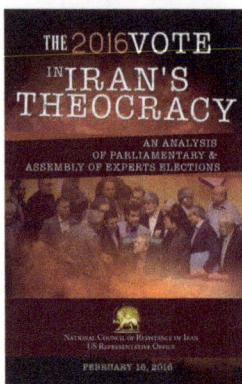

The 2016 Vote in Iran's Theocracy: An analysis of Parliamentary & Assembly of Experts Elections

February 2016, 70 pages

This book examines all the relevant data about the 2016 Assembly of Experts as well as Parliamentary elections ahead of the February 2016 elections. It looks at the history of elections since the revolution in 1979 and highlights the current intensified infighting among the various factions of the Iranian regime.

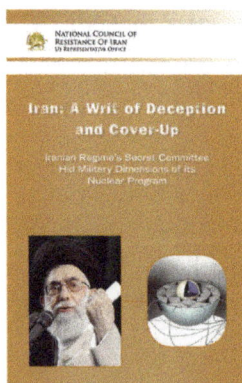

IRAN: A Writ of Deception and Cover-up: Iranian Regime's Secret Committee Hid Military Dimensions of its Nuclear Program

February 2016, 30 pages

The book provides details about a top-secret committee in charge of forging response to the International Atomic Energy Agency (IAEA) regarding the Possible Military Dimensions (PMD) of Tehran's nuclear program, including those related to the detonators called EBW (Exploding Bridge Wire), an integral part of developing an implosion type nuclear device.

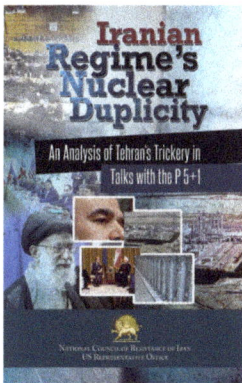

Iranian Regime's Nuclear Duplicity: An Analysis of Tehran's Trickery in Talks with the P 5+1

January 2016, 74 pages

This book examines Iran's behavior throughout the negotiations process in an effort to inform the current dialogue on a potential agreement. Drawing on both publicly available sources and those within Iran, the book focuses on two major periods of intense negotiations with the regime: 2003-2004 and 2013-2015.

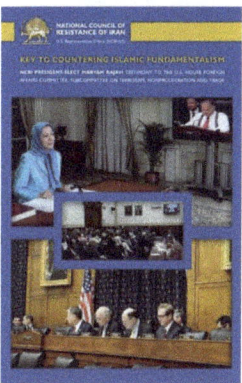

Key to Countering Islamic Fundamentalism: Maryam Rajavi? Testimony To The U.S. House Foreign Affairs Committee

June 2015, 68 pages

Testimony before U.S. House Foreign Affairs Committee's subcommittee on Terrorism, non-Proliferation, and Trade discussing ISIS and Islamic fundamentalism. The book contains Maryam Rajavi's full testimony as well as the question and answer by representatives.

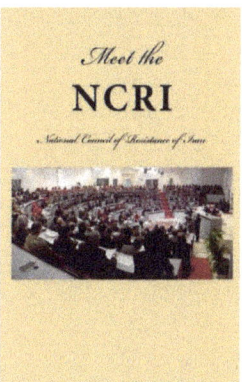

Meet the National Council of Resistance of Iran

June 2014, 150 pages

Meet the National Council of Resistance of Iran discusses what NCRI stands for, what its platform is, and why a vision for a free, democratic, secular, non-nuclear republic in Iran would serve world peace.

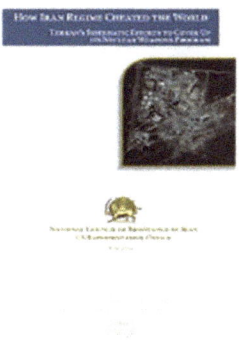

How Iran Regime Cheated the World: Tehran's Systematic Efforts to Cover Up its Nuclear Weapons Program

June 2014, 50 pages

The monograph discusses the Iranian regime's report card as far as it relates to being transparent when addressing the international community's concerns about the true nature and the ultimate purpose of its nuclear program.

About the NCRI-US

The National Council of Resistance of Iran-US Representative Office (NCRI-US) acts as the Washington office for Iran's parliament-in-exile, the National Council of Resistance of Iran, which is dedicated to the establishment of a democratic, secular, non-nuclear republic in Iran.

NCRI-US, registered as a non-profit tax-exempt organization, has been instrumental in exposing the nuclear weapons program of Iran, including the sites in Natanz, and Arak, the biological and chemical weapons program of Iran, as well as its ambitious ballistic missile program.

NCRI-US has also exposed the terrorist network of the regime, including its involvement in the bombing of Khobar Towers in Saudi Arabia, the Jewish Community Center in Argentina, its fueling of sectarian violence in Iraq and Syria, and its malign activities in other parts of the Middle East.

Our office has provided information on the human rights violations in Iran, extensive anti-government demonstrations, and the movement for democratic change in Iran.

Visit our website at www.ncrius.org

You may follow us on   **twitter**   @ncrius

Follow us on   **facebook**   NCRIUS

You can also find us on   **Instagram**   NCRIUS

www.ingramcontent.com/pod-product-compliance
Lightning Source LLC
Chambersburg PA
CBHW051311020426
42333CB00027B/3301